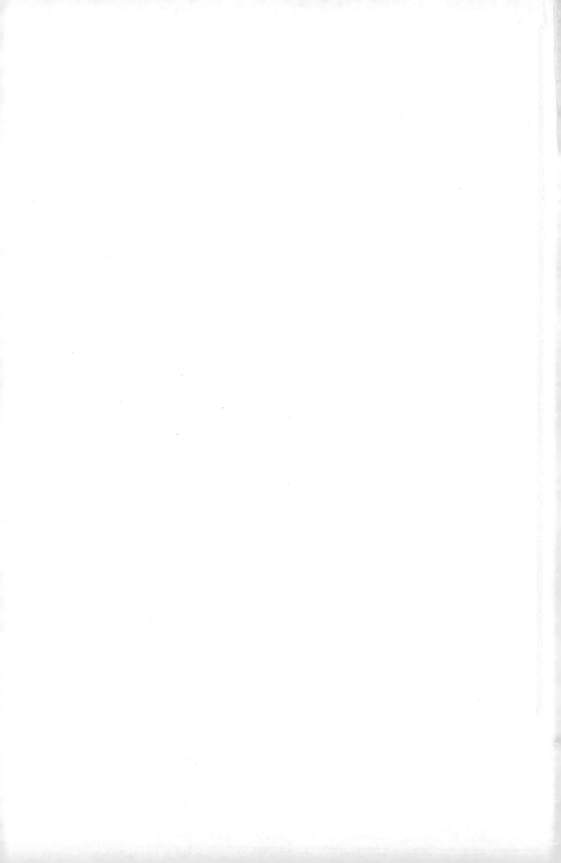

Addiction Treatment

Addiction Treatment
Science and Policy for the Twenty-first Century

EDITED BY

JACK E. HENNINGFIELD
The Johns Hopkins University School of Medicine
Baltimore, Maryland
Pinney Associates
Bethesda, Maryland

PATRICIA B. SANTORA
The Johns Hopkins University School of Medicine
Baltimore, Maryland

and

WARREN K. BICKEL
University of Arkansas for Medical Sciences
Little Rock, Arkansas

The Johns Hopkins University Press
Baltimore

© 2007 The Johns Hopkins University Press
All rights reserved. Published 2007
Printed in the United States of America on acid-free paper
9 8 7 6 5 4 3 2 1

The Johns Hopkins University Press
2715 North Charles Street
Baltimore, Maryland 21218-4363
www.press.jhu.edu

Library of Congress Cataloging-in-Publication Data

Addiction treatment : science and policy for the twenty-first century /
edited by Jack E. Henningfield, Patricia B. Santora, and Warren K. Bickel.
    p. ; cm.
  Includes bibliographical references and index.
  ISBN-13: 978-0-8018-8669-0 (hardcover : alk. paper)
  ISBN-10: 0-8018-8669-4 (hardcover : alk. paper)
  1. Substance abuse—Treatment. 2. Compulsive behavior—Social
aspects. 3. Compulsive behavior—Treatment. I. Henningfield, Jack E.
II. Santora, Patricia B., 1949–   III. Bickel, Warren K.
  [DNLM: 1. Substance-Related Disorders—therapy—United States.
2. Attitude to Health—United States. 3. Health Policy—United States.
4. Health Services Accessibility—United States. WM 270 A22428 2007]
  RA564.A3348 2007
  362.29—dc22   2006103126

A catalog record for this book is available from the British Library.

The "Introduction," by C. Everett Koop, M.D., Sc.D., was originally published in 2003 as "Drug Addiction in America: Challenges and Opportunities" in *Military Medicine* (168[5]:viii–xvi). It is reprinted here with
permission.

Contents

II.   Special Populations

Color illustrations follow page 94.

Contributors

Warren K. Bickel, Ph.D., Wilbur D. Mills Chair of Alcoholism and Drug Abuse Prevention, Professor of Psychiatry, and Director, Center for Addiction Research, University of Arkansas for Medical Sciences, Little Rock, Arkansas

H. Westley Clark, M.D., J.D., M.P.H., Director, Center for Substance Abuse Treatment, Substance Abuse and Mental Health Services Administration, Rockville, Maryland

Joseph R. DiFranza, M.D., Professor of Family Medicine and Community Health, Department of Family Medicine and Community Health, University of Massachusetts Medical School, Worcester, Massachusetts

Edward F. Domino, M.D., Professor of Pharmacology, Department of Pharmacology, University of Michigan, Ann Arbor, Michigan

Michael C. Fiore, M.D., M.P.H., Professor of Medicine and Director, Center for Tobacco Research and Intervention, University of Wisconsin School of Medicine and Public Health, Madison, Wisconsin

Larry M. Gentilello, M.D., Professor and Chairman, Division of Burns, Trauma, and Critical Care, University of Texas Southwestern Medical School, Dallas, Texas

Gary A. Giovino, Ph.D., M.S., Professor of Health Behavior, Department of Health Behavior, State University of New York at Buffalo, School of Public Health and Health Professions, Buffalo, New York; formerly Senior Research Scientist, Department of Health Behavior,

Division of Cancer Prevention and Population Sciences, Roswell Park Cancer Institute, Buffalo, New York

Jack E. Henningfield, Ph.D., Professor of Behavioral Biology, Adjunct, Department of Psychiatry and Behavioral Sciences, and Director, Innovators Combating Substance Abuse Awards Program, Johns Hopkins University School of Medicine, Baltimore, Maryland, and Vice President, Research and Health Policy, Pinney Associates, Bethesda, Maryland

Heidi E. Hutton, Ph.D., Assistant Professor, Department of Psychiatry and Behavioral Sciences, Johns Hopkins University School of Medicine, Baltimore, Maryland

Hendree Jones, Ph.D., Associate Professor, Department of Psychiatry and Behavioral Sciences, Johns Hopkins University School of Medicine, Baltimore, Maryland

C. Everett Koop, M.D., Sc.D., Elizabeth DeCamp McInerny Professor and Senior Scholar, Koop Institute, Dartmouth Medical School, Hanover, New Hampshire; Surgeon General of the United States (1982–1989); Surgeon-in-Chief, Children's Hospital of Philadelphia (1948–1981), Philadelphia, Pennsylvania

Alan I. Leshner, Ph.D., Chief Executive Officer, American Association for the Advancement of Science, Washington, D.C.

Lisa A. Marsch, Ph.D., Senior Principal Investigator, National Development and Research Institutes, Inc., New York, New York

Raymond Materson, Artist-in-Residence, Ark, Inc., Troy, New York

Jesse B. Milby, Ph.D., ABPP, Professor of Psychology, Medicine, Psychiatry, and Public Health, and Director, Medical/Clinical Psychology Doctoral Program, University of Alabama at Birmingham, Birmingham, Alabama

William R. Miller, Ph.D., Emeritus Distinguished Professor, Department of Psychology, University of New Mexico, Albuquerque, New Mexico

Eric T. Moolchan, M.D., Director, Teen Tobacco Addiction Treatment Research Clinic, Intramural Research Program, National Institute on Drug Abuse, National Institutes of Health, Baltimore, Maryland

Mark W. Parrino, M.P.A., Founder and President, American Association for the Treatment of Opioid Dependence, New York, New York

Stanton Peele, Ph.D., J.D., Senior Fellow, Drug Policy Alliance, and

Adjunct Professor, Department of Psychology, New School University, New York, New York

James O. Prochaska, Ph.D., Director, Cancer Prevention Research Center, University of Rhode Island, Providence, Rhode Island

James L. Repace, M.Sc., Visiting Assistant Professor, Department of Public Health and Family Medicine, Tufts University School of Medicine, Boston, Massachusetts, and Biophysicist, Repace Associates, Inc., Bowie, Maryland

Paul N. Samuels, J.D., President and Director, Legal Action Center, New York, New York

Patricia B. Santora, Ph.D., Assistant Professor, Department of Psychiatry and Behavioral Sciences, and Deputy Director, Innovators Combating Substance Abuse Awards Program, Johns Hopkins University School of Medicine, Baltimore, Maryland

Sally Satel, M.D., Resident Scholar, American Enterprise Institute for Public Policy Research, Washington, D.C., and Staff Psychiatrist, Oasis Drug Clinic, Washington, D.C.

Maxine L. Stitzer, Ph.D., Professor, Department of Psychiatry and Behavioral Sciences, Johns Hopkins University School of Medicine, Baltimore, Maryland

Alexander C. Wagenaar, Ph.D., Professor of Epidemiology and Health Policy Research, University of Florida, College of Medicine, Gainesville, Florida

Lawrence Wallack, Dr.P.H., Dean, College of Urban and Public Affairs, Portland State University, Portland, Oregon

Jeffrey J. Weiss, Ph.D., Assistant Professor, Department of Psychiatry, and Director, AIDS Psychiatry Research Group, Mount Sinai School of Medicine, New York, New York

Robert West, Ph.D., B.Sc., Professor of Health Psychology, Cancer Research United Kingdom Health Behaviour Unit, Department of Epidemiology and Public Health, University College London, England

Curtis Wright, M.D., M.P.H., Vice President, Risk Management and Regulatory Affairs, Javelin Pharmaceuticals, Cambridge, Massachusetts

Preface

JACK E. HENNINGFIELD, PH.D.,
PATRICIA B. SANTORA, PH.D., AND
WARREN K. BICKEL, PH.D.

Substance abuse and addiction to alcohol, tobacco, illicit drugs, and prescription drugs account for approximately one in five deaths in the United States, or more than one-half million persons each year (Mokdad et al., 2004). The economic effects of substance abuse and addiction are enormous: the combined costs of health care, lost productivity, crime, and so forth have been estimated at well over one-half trillion U.S. dollars, with approximately $185 billion for illicit drug abuse (Office of National Drug Control Policy, 2004), $180 billion for alcohol abuse and dependence (Mark et al., 2005), and $170 billion for tobacco dependence (*MMWR*, 2005). As staggering as these costs may be, they tell only part of the story. Financial costs do not reflect the suffering of too many families that have watched in anguish as a loved one struggled with addiction.

Many have experienced the enormous frustration of suspecting that treatment was available but learning that it was out of reach or unacceptable to the person in need. Those of us involved in substance abuse research, treatment, and policy share this grief, and our frustration may be even greater because we know that much more is possible when treatment is made readily available. This is not to say that we have all the answers; we do not. Like medical providers in the early days of penicillin, we have the knowledge and ability to save many lives even as we recognize the limitations of current therapies. Whereas few questioned the importance of improving antibiotics and making them as accessible as possible, today people debate the value of seeking to improve treatment for addiction or assuring that those who need treatment have access to it.

We *do* have effective treatments for many forms of drug addiction, and such treatments enable millions of individuals to live, function, and contribute to society, but we do not yet have effective therapy for all forms of addiction or for every substance abuser or addicted person. Rather than accelerate the quest for better treatments, however, the limitations of today's treatments have led some to question the importance of treatment in addressing substance abuse. Many conclude that the problem is not with the treatments but with the substance abusers and addicted individuals who will not accept the treatments or who refuse to heal themselves. In actuality, McLellan and colleagues (2000) showed that addiction treatment is comparable to treatment for asthma, hypertension, or diabetes when measures such as compliance with treatment demands and relapse to disease symptoms were reviewed. Major differences in attitudes and treatment approaches, however, are noteworthy. When treating most medical conditions, health professionals will explore several treatment options with the patient to determine which is acceptable and effective (McLellan, 2002), whereas with addiction treatment a person is typically offered a single option in a "one-size-fits-all" approach that fails for many.

Research into drug addiction is addressing the challenge of building the scientific foundation for more effective and acceptable treatments. Health care providers and policymakers arguably face an even greater challenge of ensuring that effective treatments are available to those who need them and of devising systems to disseminate innovative treatments for substance abuse as rapidly as innovations in other areas of medical care.

Consider HIV/AIDS. Two decades ago it was considered a death sentence, with no treatment available and skepticism that treatment was even possible. Research institutions, policymakers, the U.S. Food and Drug Administration, pharmaceutical companies, scientists, and many others rallied, perhaps not always on the same path but generally pursuing the same goal. Leaders such as former Surgeon General C. Everett Koop made clear that we should be fighting the disease and not those afflicted. Within ten years, promising treatments began to emerge, and today millions of HIV-infected individuals live productive and fulfilling lives. Some of the same challenges, such as access to treatment and limited efficacy and tolerability, face those who have addictive disorders. These challenges include the stigma carried by those with drug abuse and addiction disorders, limited access to and effectiveness of treatment, and the fact that people are often offered a treatment modality that is not acceptable and then blamed for failing to comply with its demands.

We conceived this book to help revolutionize and energize debate and discussion about what the treatment of drug addiction in the United States should look like. We asked leading thinkers from many disciplines in the addiction field to offer their perspectives on what addiction treatment could and should look like as we progress into the twenty-first century. Many of these contributors have been recognized as innovators by their peers and by society. They include men and women who have been at the forefront of basic research in addiction, health care providers with expertise in treating special populations and problems, policymakers, legal experts, and visual artists. We challenged them to be creative and constructive by writing focused chapters, not technical review articles, in their own voices. We encouraged them to explore novel, promising, and, in some cases, provocative aspects of addiction treatment. All of the contributors have fascinating things to say, and we find their diversity in ideas and style invigorating. Visual artists with personal experience in substance abuse and addiction also provide insights into the human dimension of addiction and recovery that complement the scientific perspective.

We believe the book will be useful to students and professionals, other thought leaders, and those who are interested in but have little training in addiction science or treatment. We begin with an introduction by former Surgeon General C. Everett Koop, one of America's most thoughtful and innovative health care leaders ever. Broad in its scope, this chapter is based on a keynote address Dr. Koop gave at the National Press Club in February 2003, in which he outlined the key issues, controversies, challenges, and opportunities facing the field of substance abuse and addiction (Koop, 2003). His vision of what could be possible if addiction were addressed more as a public health challenge than as a "war to be won" provided a stimulus for many of the authors contributing to this book. The subsequent chapters are relatively brief and are more specifically focused on one or another aspect of addiction highlighted by Dr. Koop.

The book consists of three parts. Part I examines the emerging science and theoretical thinking that underlie the development of treatment models. It provides the foundation on which the remaining two sections are built. The first part of the book explores the essence of addiction as a disorder of self-control that is modulated and perpetuated by chemical, physiological, behavioral, and social forces. Drug types include alcohol, tobacco, stimulant and sedative drugs, and others, and, although each drug category poses unique challenges, many of the observations and lessons can apply to all drug classes. Also discussed in this section are implications for other treatment models that might be more broadly incorporated into general health settings, extended by computer-based treatment and education, and magnified by state-of-the-art behavioral approaches.

Many discussions of addiction treatment fail to address the numerous challenges experienced by various populations in specific life circumstances (e.g., pregnancy, adolescence, those with multiple medical conditions, etc.). These "special populations" are featured in part II, which emphasizes the importance of ensuring that addiction treatment solutions meant to address the needs of one population do not inadvertently harm other populations. In some cases, past "solutions" have been counterproductive. For example, legal sanctions can be the path to addiction treatment for those who are incarcerated, but they can be a deadly roadblock for pregnant women who use intravenous drugs and do not seek prenatal care for fear they will lose their babies to protective services. The enormous numbers of substance-abusing persons who have other concurrent diseases, including HIV/AIDS and psychiatric disorders, that significantly complicate addiction treatment create additional challenges. Examples of addiction art explore the human side of addiction through the lenses of visual artists' stunning insights into addiction and recovery.

Part III explores numerous health care, social, and policy issues that challenge our views about addiction and its treatment. This section includes lively debate on current topics ranging from basic attitudes and conceptions about substance abuse and addiction, to issues of privacy and discrimination, to legislation for broad-based public health policies. Some of the views posed are radically at odds with those expressed by other contributors to this book, but they are based on insights that cannot be ignored and reflect beliefs that are too widespread to be dismissed. Compounding the challenges to treatment innovation and access is the fact that addictive drug use can be marketed and enabled by economic forces. As broad as the challenges are, the potential solutions are even broader, including more innovative approaches by the Food and Drug Administration, general health care providers, and even dietitians.

We hope that, for the policymaker, researcher, health professional, addicted person, or concerned friend of a substance abuser, this volume will be engaging and will stimulate further thinking. Our hope is that readers will not only enjoy learning what some of the most creative thinkers in the field have to say about addiction and its treatment but also find themselves thinking differently about addiction treatment and making their own contributions from their personal spheres of interest and influence.

REFERENCES

Koop, C.E. 2003. Drug addiction in America: challenges and opportunities (special feature). *Military Medicine* 168:viii–xvi.

Mark, T.L., Coffey, R.M., McKusick, D.R., Harwood, H., Bouchery, E., Genuardi, J., Vandivort, R., Buch, J., and Dilonardo, J. 2005. *National Estimates of Expenditures for Mental Health Services and Substance Abuse Treatment, 1991–2001.* SAMHSA Publication No. SMA 05-3999. Rockville, Md.: Substance Abuse and Mental Health Services Administration.

McLellan, A.T. 2002. Have we evaluated addiction treatment correctly? Implications from a chronic care perspective. *Addiction* 97:249–52.

McLellan, A.T., Lewis, D.C., O'Brien, C.P., and Kleber, H.D. 2000. Drug dependence, a chronic medical illness: implications for treatment, insurance, and outcomes evaluation. *JAMA* 284:1689–95.

MMWR. 2005. Annual Smoking-Attributable Mortality, Years of Potential Life Lost, and Productivity Losses, United States, 1997–2001. 54, no. 25 (July 1):625–28.

Mokdad, A.H., Marks, J.S., Stroup, D.F., and Gerberding, J.L. 2004. Actual causes of death in the United States, 2000. *JAMA* 291:1238–45.

Office of National Drug Control Policy. 2004. *The Economic Costs of Drug Abuse in the United States, 1992–2002.* Publication no. 207303. Washington, D.C.: Executive Office of the President.

Introduction
Drug Addiction in America: Challenges and Opportunities

C. EVERETT KOOP, M.D., SC.D.

I would like to cover the subject of drug addiction in America as the dew covers the ground. I hope that you will use my comments as a compass to find your way through this complex public health problem—one that cannot be solved by simplistic "solutions" embodied in such catchphrases as "legalization" and "medicalization"—to the end that we find some solid guideposts.

First, the keystone of the world of addiction is addiction to the legal substance tobacco because of its addictive ingredient, nicotine. Tobacco is a major risk factor in adolescents for getting drunk and using marijuana. The goal of the tobacco industry is to addict as many people as early as possible. Everything else big tobacco does is "theater." Because of the annual number of deaths worldwide, because of the economic implications of addiction, disease, disability, and death worldwide, and because the primary target is children worldwide, the entire enterprise of big tobacco is the largest concentration of evil masquerading as a legitimate business on this planet.

Second, there is no court of appeal because the lawmakers who could change the situation will not act—they are supported too heavily financially by the tobacco industry.

Third, stick to public health in an effort that is supported by *appropriate* measures to reduce supply, understanding that the problem will not be controlled by overly focusing on the supply side. The word *appropriate* is one of two words essential to success; the other is *flexible*.

Unfortunately, both words have been dropped from Washington's legislative and bureaucratic vocabularies.

Fourth, it is easy to get addictive drugs, but it is difficult for most folks who need it to get treatment. One night in Denver, I was told by a young man that, in an unfamiliar city, he could purchase cocaine within twenty minutes. He proved to be right, and I've learned that the solution to drug addiction won't come until it is as easy to find treatment for drug addiction as it is to find addictive drugs.

Fifth, our national philosophy should be as finely tuned to getting treatment as is the system for interdicting drug runners.

Sixth, drug addiction is a disease. Whether you are concerned with tobacco, alcohol, or street drugs, it is more than just a brain disease; it involves social, economic, and psychological elements that must be addressed. In addition, what may work for one culture may not be appropriate for another. (There's that word again.) For example, drug addiction is strongly influenced by social forces, which can result in relatively low levels of tobacco consumption in states such as Utah and California but much higher levels in states such as Kentucky and Virginia.

Drug addiction can be strongly altered by such factors as the cost and availability of the drug in question. We saw this when the drug cocaine went from being thought of as a relatively nonaddictive drug in the 1970s to becoming the flagship of addiction in the 1980s. It became cheap and available, and that epidemic emerged in the early 1980s even before "crack" cocaine became generally available.

This brings me to the physical form of some of the drugs in question. From the public health perspective, cocaine got even worse when it became more like cigarettes than like a forbidden street drug, when it could be sold in relatively inexpensive doses in a form that could mimic the rush effects of an injection by the simple act of smoking the drug. Wine coolers placed next to soft drinks in supermarkets do not make alcohol more addictive. They make alcohol more acceptable and easier for adolescents to consume.

Marijuana is widely considered to be nonaddicting by people who do not realize that its potential is constrained only by the limitation on its availability. Would a person in favor of legalizing marijuana want his commercial airline pilot or his surgeon smoking marijuana? Members of congressional committees held the misconception that, if one ever kicked the habit, that person had not been addicted. How could nicotine be addictive, they argued, when so many people stop smoking? Education on addiction can never stop.

Seventh, we must show compassion for those afflicted with addictions and help them with the same passion we reserve for others who are sick and injured. Moral and criminal aspects are also prominent in the sale of illicit drugs or, for that matter, in the deplorable marketing to children and adolescents by tobacco companies to provide the pipeline of new smokers needed to replace those being killed by their products. I'm referring to compassion for the addicted person, not compassion for the drug lord or the tobacco executive, who are motivated only by greed and have already abrogated any sense of personal responsibility. What is the difference between a drug lord in Colombia, his lieutenant in Miami, or an executive of a cigarette company? None. They are all evil; I would gladly spend the rest of my life bringing them to their knees, where, I confess, I would deal with them without mercy.

And then we have prescription drugs, for which control mechanisms are intended to strike the right balance between enabling appropriate (there's that word again) patient access and reducing diversion and abuse. If the right balance is not struck, patients in need may suffer while abuse continues. There are numerous examples in which overzealous government agents bent on eliminating all addictive drugs from the marketplace have run roughshod over palliative care. What, then, is the right message concerning prescription drugs? Certainly not that analgesics, for example, are bad. Morphine and its analogues are not only among the most addictive of all drugs but are also the most effective drugs for people with intractable pain. On the appropriate use of morphine hang several ethical issues, such as assisted suicide, euthanasia, and so on. Thus, an appropriate and flexible attitude toward the use of palliative drugs for pain is essential if we are to sustain ethical practice in palliative medicine.

Eighth, fight the disease of addiction and the purveyors of disease, not those afflicted. One of the most important sentences I ever wrote was when I rightly said (in the report on acquired immunodeficiency syndrome that President Reagan asked me to write for the American people): "We are fighting a disease and not the people who have it." Today, also, we are not fighting the victims of addiction; we are fighting the disease that causes their problem. Too often blame is laid on those with addictions as though they sought and intended to become addicted. Perhaps they did make poor choices about drug use, but all too frequently the choice was made during adolescence or earlier. That is not the same thing as having decided to abuse *and* become addicted to drugs.

My own studies entirely convinced me that most adolescents—like congressional representatives—understand little about the nature of addiction. Adolescents may talk about tobacco as "addicting," but they are *completely* confident that such would never happen to them because they would never let it happen to them. Addiction doesn't come heralded by a brass band; it sneaks up, sometimes with extraordinary rapidity.

The picture becomes more complex when we consider the vast differences among drugs in terms of the nature of their addictive and damaging effects. For example, in the case of alcohol, the damage and harm range from violence, false courage, poor judgment, and drunk-driving homicides to liver cirrhosis that may develop in heavy drinkers. Yet the evidence is also clear that appropriate amounts of alcohol and appropriate frequency can provide benefits in terms of reducing the risk of heart attacks.

In the case of heroin, however, some deaths are caused by overdosing on the drug itself, but most of the tragedies associated with heroin are the results of side effects of the addiction: the sharing of drug paraphernalia for taking it intravenously that transmits HIV/AIDS or hepatitis—sharing that is very much a part of the culture of intravenous drug abuse.

With cocaine, the lucrative and highly competitive trade itself has become a source of deadly violence, augmented by overly aggressive actions that are part of the body's physiologic response to high doses of cocaine.

Nicotine is addicting, but it does not cause cancer, nor for that matter is it considered a major factor in most tobacco-caused disease. Recent media misinterpretations of research from the National Cancer Institute concerning nicotine and lung cancer were not only incorrect but also a disservice to smokers who are trying to quit using nicotine patches or gum.

One of the highlights of my tenure as surgeon general was the release of the surgeon general's report *The Health Consequences of Smoking: Nicotine Addiction* in 1988 (U.S. Department of Health and Human Services, 1988). Big tobacco denied the science and truth of that report, but subsequent disclosures of once secret documents revealed that the industry knew much more about the addictive nature of nicotine than did the federal government and knew it decades earlier. And can we ever forget the chief executive officers of the major tobacco companies lying individually under oath before a congressional committee in 1990, that they "didn't believe nicotine was addictive"?

More than once when testifying before a congressional committee I was asked, if nicotine is as addictive as I said it was, why aren't people shooting one another in order to get it? My answer was simple: "Remove nicotine from society, and you will see the same behavior that you see in reference to cocaine." Another frequently asked question was, "If tobacco is as dangerous as you say it is, why don't you take it off the market?" The answer? "With close to 50 million folks addicted to nicotine in this country, it would be not only inhumane, but also unmanageable to remove the fix from so many people. That's why the Food and Drug Administration (FDA), an arm of the U.S. Public Health Service, would never suddenly abolish tobacco or remove nicotine from tobacco products."

Ninth, and last, we need innovation in education, prevention, treatment, and policy. The vagaries of addiction, like a mutating virus, force us to alter our strategies with equal speed.

As I have grown older, I have come to realize that clichés I have used might actually be detrimental to my overall goals in public health. A statement used by many people who are in the business of tobacco control is "smoking kills." If we just talk about death from tobacco, we leave out all the dreadful things that precede death, such as sickness and disability. I rather have the feeling that if I were suffering from chronic obstructive lung disease, I would view death as a friend and not an enemy.

Also, I think I have been wrong in using "war" as a metaphor in discussing tobacco. We speak of the "tobacco wars," we use words such as "battlefield," "enemy," "fight against evil," and so forth. Now, I know that in a sense we *are* at war against the tobacco industry, against the drug lords, their distributors, and their pushers, but if we begin to think that this is the kind of a war that can be won like a military war, or that we can eradicate addiction as we eradicated smallpox, we are certainly doomed to fail even though the sweet smell of success sometimes accompanies our rhetoric. If we are going to use a metaphor of war, perhaps one associated with terrorism is a better choice in which the enemy is constantly moving, changing his tactics, attacking from within and without and from unexpected places, which leaves us with no single target to get in our sights.

We have to be careful with disease metaphors as well. We are certainly not dealing with smallpox; we are dealing with something much more like HIV/AIDS, where the forces that cause the spread of the problem are many and diverse while the obstacles to appropriate action are caused more by indifference and prejudice than they are by the disease process itself.

I was surgeon general when the AIDS epidemic first became apparent. Public health actions were inhibited because we were dealing with a *political* disease of great complexity. Public health actions were precluded by the views of some that HIV/AIDS would run its course in homosexuals and in intravenous drug abusers—and, after all, didn't they deserve what they got? I was the surgeon general of all the people in the United States and one who cared about *all* the people and who also understood that there was no such thing as a disease that would keep itself confined to one or two socially identifiable and—at the moment—despised populations. AIDS brought something new to American medicine, and it has strong implications for our concern about addiction. In the early stages of the AIDS epidemic, for the first time in American history, we saw health professionals withholding their expertise from people because they didn't like the process by which those patients became ill.

Being as close to the epidemic of AIDS, as I was, and filling the role of spokesperson for the government to the public on AIDS, I am proud of the work of the public health community and how much was accomplished in this area of medicine. I wish I could be as proud of our fight against addiction. HIV/AIDS and nicotine addiction are similar in that, with proper treatment and by dealing with them as the public health menace that they are, we can offer individuals the opportunity to live out their normal life expectancies. We have a long way to go, in both treatment and prevention. Above all, there is no such concept as a disease that is someone else's problem.

Addiction is a *global* tragedy. Tobacco carries the same global implication as HIV/AIDS. What has happened to the global conscience? How can we countenance the fact that 500 million people alive now on the planet will die prematurely in the next *twenty-five* years? If that's too big a number to take in, let's talk about my small state of

New Hampshire. Thirty-four thousand children now alive in New Hampshire will die prematurely from tobacco. Where is the outrage?

Having said that addiction in America is a terribly complex problem that cannot be dealt with simplistically, I am not going to say that I have the answer in the form of a simple solution. My suggestion is to treat drug addiction as the controllable public health problem it actually is and that the common sense use of appropriate, flexible, proven measures of control focused on public health is adequate to address the diverse problems we face today. Perhaps we do not even understand the drug types and social behavior surrounding drug abuse that will be our headaches of tomorrow.

What if we applied comprehensive public health approaches to the control of drug addiction?

What if we recognized that a person could develop an addiction to a drug even as he or she can develop diseases such as liver cirrhosis from alcoholism or lung cancer from cigarette smoking?

Suppose we relieved the Coast Guard of the task of chasing drug runners through the Caribbean and let them return to their chartered obligation of protecting our coasts?

What if we brought a better balance to efforts to reduce supply and demand by increasing our ability to help those afflicted with addiction so that they would not perpetuate the cycle in themselves and pass it on to others?

Suppose I could have told the young man in Denver who bragged about being able to find cocaine in twenty minutes that I could find help for him by calling the equivalent of a 911 number—perhaps 811?

If we really believe everything we know to be true about tobacco addiction and understand it as a serious, preventable risk factor for other forms of drug and alcohol abuse, why have we never had a drug czar who took seriously the public health burden of the abuse of legal drugs like tobacco and alcohol instead of concentrating solely on illicit drugs?

What if the secretary of health and human services wanted to make the treatment of addiction a comprehensive and coordinated goal of the U.S. Public Health Service?

The National Institutes of Health could increase funding of research efforts aimed at addiction, and the FDA could put any medications resulting from such research on a fast track (as they did for medications of possible benefit to HIV/AIDS). What if the Public Health

Service began to talk more regularly with the Drug Enforcement Administration?

What if the White House instructed the drug czar to stop chasing smugglers' boats in the Gulf of Mexico and instead to make sure that emerging treatments were not so restricted that using them to treat addiction would be a practical impossibility?

In 2002, the FDA approved a new treatment for heroin addiction—buprenorphine. This treatment is as effective as methadone and offers advantages for at least some people who are either receiving methadone or for whom methadone is unacceptable or unavailable. As important as is the medicine itself is the fact that people in need can get it in a doctor's office, provided the doctor has received necessary training, patients do not need to go to a methadone clinic that might be inaccessible or inappropriate under their circumstance. This treatment avenue demonstrated the importance of many parties working together. The road was paved by scientists in the public and private sector who developed the drug, but the door to more accessible treatment was opened by congressional legislation—the Drug Abuse Treatment Act of 2000 (or, DATA 2000). It was supported by both major parties in Congress and the Oval Office, as well as the Departments of Justice and Health and Human Services, so this drug will be made available through doctors' offices across the country; it is a minor inconvenience that physicians who choose to prescribe it will need special certification. The important thing is that this medication will finally make treatment available in places like Denver, where street drugs are as accessible as my young friend proved but where treatment is still an unattainable dream.

Let me give an example of how public health can work and why public health does not mean only "either/or" when it comes to policy or reducing supply or demand. During the 1970s, when state after state lowered its minimum age for procuring alcohol to 18 or 19, highway deaths among young people soared. In response, many states raised alcohol procurement age to 21. Scientists documented that, as these age levels were increased in the context of other public health efforts, including education, the highway death count began to decline in state after state, with some of the most pronounced effects among the young. In essence, this was a grim experiment in national drug control policy, but one we should learn from and take to heart.

Because of the strong benefits of these efforts, during the 1980s, the federal government encouraged states to raise the minimum purchase age for alcohol beverages to 21, to reduce the blood alcohol concentration used to define "driving while intoxicated," to take measures to educate the public more effectively about the dangers of drinking and driving, and to encourage more aggressive efforts to get drunk drivers off the highways.

In 1988, during National Drunk and Drugged Driving Prevention Month (December), just before the holidays, I organized an invitational surgeon general's workshop on drunk driving. The Brewers of America joined with the Vintners of America in going before federal court to get an injunction prohibiting me from having such a conference. How could anyone be against drunk driving? Fortunately, the alcohol industry lost, we held the workshop, and the participants were reenergized by the effort of the industry. The supporting coalition was broad and included scientists, voluntary organizations, such as Mothers against Drunk Driving, the U.S. Department of Transportation, law enforcement organizations, and the Reagan administration. Workshop participants went home and pursued aggressively the recommendations to further strengthen laws and other efforts to reduce drunk driving.

Let me give another example. During the 1980s, cigarette smoking among adult Americans seemed to have become stuck at about 25 percent of the population. By the early 1990s, smoking among youth began to increase dramatically as cigarettes began to be promoted more effectively to this population and their relative price dropped so low as to make this an addiction even young people could afford.

In the past three years, with increased cigarette prices caused by increased taxes and tobacco litigation payments, with increased anti-tobacco campaigns from groups such as the American Legacy Foundation, with the tobacco control efforts of such states as Massachusetts and California, with increased restrictions on workplace and public smoking, and with the increased availability of treatment as well as advertising to stimulate cessation, smoking in all populations has decreased, with the greatest declines among the young. Please remember that progress is not the total elimination of addiction, it is the reduction of addiction.

Here is another example, one that did not take place on my watch. Some may not know that Richard Nixon was involved in more than one war, as he put it, and the lesser-known war was on drugs. The

Nixon administration performed an experiment that we can learn from today.

When the administration realized that there were potentially tens of thousands of heroin-addicted soldiers among returning Vietnam veterans who might soon be flooding the streets and spreading the crime and devastation assumed to be intrinsic to addiction, Nixon recognized that something had to be done.

The army began the experiment with perhaps the most radical proposal of all. Without legalizing the drugs, the army decided that soldiers who were identified as drug users would not face legal sanctions but would be treated. It then set a simple goal across the nation: to make every effort to ensure that wherever there was addiction access to treatment would be available for all.

Within three years of their return to the United States, 90 percent of the former heroin-using soldiers were clean, and cities that achieved the most dramatic *increases* in treatment access were rewarded with dramatic *decreases* of violent and drug-associated crime. This shows that drug addiction can be modified by a variety of factors and we need to do a better job controlling them.

Following the September 11 terrorist attack on New York City and Washington, D.C., many local, state and national government officials attempted to reassure their citizens by telling them what they could do to protect themselves and their communities from further harm. It was about a week following the attack that the mayor of Baltimore, Martin O'Malley, was asked what people could do to protect themselves. He answered, "To protect yourselves from harm, the most important things you can do are to wear your seatbelts, don't drink and drive, and don't smoke."

I don't think anyone thought he was trivializing terrorist threats, but it was an important reminder to keep things in perspective, a reminder that on a daily basis these are among the most important things people can do to protect themselves and families from harm. Perhaps he had in mind the apparent absurdity of the cigarette smoker purchasing an expensive gas mask to save his life, the chance of one in several millions, while he faces a one in two chance that devastating illness from that cigarette will prematurely end his life.

Many youth on the road to chronic drug abuse and addiction may be helped if they are reached earlier by members of their own communities, their churches, their schools, and their families. It is clear that youth often respond more strongly to what their parents do than to what their parents say. But that doesn't keep me from saying something to parents: "If you want to make a difference in contributing to the reduction of drug addiction and abuse in America, start by setting a good example. Don't use tobacco or drink to excess. And I hope that it is obvious that you should not be abusing marijuana or other illicit drugs, or prescription drugs, yourself."

The children of nonsmoking parents are about half as likely to smoke as the children of smoking parents. Also, nonsmoking children are many times less likely to get drunk or to smoke marijuana or use other addictive drugs. These are facts. Recent data show that, when smoking parents of smoking children quit, their children in turn are twice as likely to quit.

Will smoking or reduced smoking by adults eliminate addiction in America? Of course not. But not smoking and quitting smoking by adults will contribute to reducing addiction in America. Simply stated, if you care about illicit drug use and drunkenness, you should care about tobacco use because it is a high risk factor.

Eventually someone will ask whether tobacco is a gateway to other addictions. What the facts show is that use of smokeless tobacco or cigarettes by adolescents is a major risk factor for getting drunk and using marijuana. That obviously means it is a *preventable* risk factor. That is why I believe that efforts to reduce smoking should not be seen as isolated efforts to reduce tobacco-caused cancer and heart disease, but, rather, it should be seen as part of our nation's overall efforts to reduce addiction and to improve health in general.

If tobacco is a major risk factor for adolescents using marijuana, what is the risk of marijuana? The authors of a paper in *JAMA* entitled "The Escalation of Drug Use in Early-Onset Cannabis Users vs. Co-Twin Controls" (Lynskey et al., 2003) concluded that the association between early cannabis use and later drug use and abuse/dependence may arise from the effects of peer and social context within which the cannabis is used and obtained. In particular, early access to cannabis may reduce perceived barriers against the use of other illegal drugs and provide access to these drugs.

When I spoke before the American Lung Association and the American Thoracic Society in Miami in 1984—and gave a speech that I had deliberately neglected to pass before the watchful eye of the Office of Management and Budget and the White House—I proposed that it was not impossible to look forward to a smoke-free society in the United States by the year 2000. I was particularly interested in graduating a smoke-free class from high school in the year 2000. I remember standing at that lectern and asking—almost demanding—that certain organizations put their shoulder to the wheel and help me in this effort.

I called specifically on organizations, such as the American Lung Association, the American Heart Association, and the American Cancer Society. I called on the Boy Scouts and Girls Scouts, the Campfire Girls, respiratory therapists, pediatricians, obstetricians, and gynecologists. There was almost no one that I didn't think had a role in leading us into a position where we might see major progress in getting rid of the scourge of tobacco.

So what can individuals and organizations do if they truly wish to be part of this public health approach to the reduction of addiction? Each can examine the importance of substance abuse and addiction in their area of activity to devise ways that they can make a difference. For example, in nearly every area of medicine and at almost every medical care facility, the presenting patients are more likely to have problems associated with drug use than those who do not need medical care. Substance abuse is often a complicating factor in their condition, yet it is often ignored. Consider that: children with asthma are exposed to smoke in their households, perhaps their pediatricians should help their parents to quit smoking for the health of the children who are their primary patients. Persons with anxiety and depression are more likely to smoke cigarettes and abuse alcohol than other patients; they should be asked about drug use and offered encouragement and assistance. People with fractures where healing might be slowed down by smoking should be counseled to quit.

And then there are emergency and trauma centers, which are deluged, often beyond their professional and financial capacity, with the victims of accidents and injuries resulting from drug and alcohol use. Studies show that offering these patients assistance can significantly reduce their drug use, and their odds of returning to the trauma center, saving both lives and limited fiscal resources. Can any emergency room or trauma center be truly state of the art if it does not have the capacity to at least diagnose drug and alcohol problems, offer basic guidance, and make referrals?

Health professionals are going to be the best that they can be in their specialty only when they know enough about addiction to identify it and refer their patients for more specialized help as indicated. But they do need to understand they can make a difference by sending unambiguous, personalized messages to their patients, such as, "Your smoking means that you have a one in two chance of becoming very sick and dying prematurely, and I strongly advise you to quit." Or, "If you drink more than one to two drinks a day, you are putting yourself at risk of life threatening liver disease and may be slipping down a path to dependence without even realizing it."

In the twenty-first century, in all areas of medicine, diagnosing and treating substance abuse and addiction should be as fundamental as advice to get sufficient exercise and eat right.

Let me come back to where I started and repeat that addiction is a disease; it is a brain disease. That is not just my idea; this is recognized by all leading medical and health authorities. Drugs of addiction physically affect the brain. They alter its structure and function. Scientists can even measure brain function, using electroencelphalographic and brain imaging techniques, to see areas of the brain responding to drug administration and withdrawal.

Cigarette withdrawal can include a dysfunction of the brain so important that the inability to concentrate by many abstinent smokers is a real physiological effect. It can be treated with medications such as nicotine gum and patches. Similarly, heroin addiction can be treated with methadone, buprenorphine, and by other means.

"But don't many people quit without treatment?" you ask. Of course, just as many people recover from streptococcal infections without antibiotics; but I hope you also know that many people have died needlessly from such infections because they did not receive treatment.

You might then ask, "Doesn't calling addiction a disease get people off the hook and take away their responsibility?" The answer is no. Nevertheless, we need to strike the right, delicate balance between holding people responsible for their behavior and working to identify and address the driving forces behind it. This is not unique to drug addiction. Giving a patient a pharmaceutical should not imply that the patient has no further role in his or her recovery.

It would be considered irresponsible to withhold medication from a patient with diabetes or hypertension if they were not adhering to their dietary plan, yet in some addiction treatment settings treatment may be withheld if the patient does not meet the standards for compliance set by that clinic.

Far be it from me to say that there should be no effort to use treatment to inspire compliance with all aspects of treatment, but I am saying that the first goal should be to help the person to achieve and sustain abstinence, and appropriate and flexible treatment should be the standard. For hypertension, diabetes, depression, and many other disorders, the expected standard of care is to offer what seems to be the most appropriate treatment, to follow the patient's progress and then change the treatment if it is not working—not to blame the patient and make no effort to accommodate the needs of the patient as is all too common in substance abuse.

I just raised a question about whether calling addiction a disease might not lead individuals to abrogate personal responsibility. I am at the beginning of what I think will be my last undertaking in this life. (No pun intended.)

I am putting together an archive with the National Library of Medicine and the Baker Library at Dartmouth of my personal interactions with the world of public health. It will be available on the Internet without cost, but it is an awesome task. My lectures alone fill 199 three-ring binders, many four inches thick. In these volumes, I came across a bit of nostalgia when I found a lecture that I gave repeatedly in 1982, on the occasions when President Reagan asked me to come over to the old Executive Office Building and talk to one group or another on some of his "pet" stands and legislative plans. It really wasn't a lecture but a series of talking points. I probably never gave them all at any one sitting, but I used many of them many times.

The lecture has no name, but those who helped me with my speeches gave it a title, which was "A Really Terrific Sermon." To talk of personal responsibility leads me to leave you with an idea—it is "a really terrific sermon."

I think that a tremendous number of the ills of our society are caused by greed and/or the abrogation of personal responsibility. I would like you to take away the thought that the addiction of the individual to a drug is not ever that individual's choice. Because of the addictive nature of the drugs in question, it really cannot be attributed solely to the abrogation of personal responsibility.

Of all the individuals and organizations I have mentioned in passing, however, which exhibit the abrogation of personal responsibility to the highest degree? It is the drug lords and their chains of command right down to the pusher. It is the decision makers in the world of big tobacco and this abrogation of personal responsibility is made all the more onerous because it is fueled only by greed.

Whatever we think of the leeches who suck the life out of our young people, we must not let our zeal to reduce the supply of drugs lure us into forgetting those who have become addicted and who create a demand for addictive drugs. We must expand greatly our efforts to help those with addictions so that getting treatment will be as easy as getting addictive drugs. When the demand is reduced, so will be the supply.

As we proceed in the twenty-first century, we should carefully consider the many lessons of the twentieth century, both positive and negative. We should build on the advances and successes: we should strive to a future in which substance abuse and addiction are minimized and a future in which people who become afflicted by drugs, including tobacco and alcohol, are treated with compassion and the best that medicine has to offer regardless of their financial means or position in society. Of course, we must be forever vigilant for new types of substance abuse that are sure to emerge and our science must keep pace. Policymakers must be adept, responding to changing societal needs with appropriate laws. Educators must ensure that the young have the tools to protect their health. Leaders must lead by example as well as by word. Doctors and other health professionals must be as willing to treat drug addiction as they are to treat other common diseases, including knowing when to refer special cases to specialists as indicated. In short, we must all work together to reduce the drug-driven plagues of the twentieth century to that of diseases such as tuberculosis, polio, and HIV, all of which seemed insurmountable at times but all of which have proved possible to control. It is a mighty challenge, but it is our opportunity to serve future generations.

REFERENCES

Lynskey, M. T., Heath, A. C., Bucholz, K. K., Slutske, W. S., Madden, P. A., Nelson, E. C., Statham, D. J., and Martin, N. G. 2003. Escalation of drug use in early-onset cannabis users vs. co-twin control. *JAMA* 289:427–33.

U.S. Department of Health and Human Services, Public Health Service. 1988. *The Health Consequences of Smoking: Nicotine Addiction. A Surgeon General's Report.* Rockville, Md.: Department of Health and Human Services.

I

Treatment Models and Emerging Science

1

Is Addiction a Problem of Self-Control?

WILLIAM R. MILLER, PH.D.

There are at least two major and seemingly divergent views of addiction in America. The older of the two regards excessive drinking and illicit drug use as willful behavior, a choice for which the individual is ultimately responsible. The Reagan-era "Just Say No" campaign is a quintessential expression of this perspective. Judicial systems commonly behave as if addictive behavior is volitional. We hold people responsible for driving under the influence (DUI) and its consequences regardless of whether they are judged to be addicted. With an informative exception, the influence of alcohol or illicit drugs is not considered a mitigating factor in violent or property crime. That exception involves offenses (other than DUI) in which the ability to form the intention to commit the crime is a pertinent factor in determining guilt. In such cases, the offender can be judged not guilty if the defense can show that he or she was incapable of forming the intention and plan to carry out the act. Moreover, defining the use of certain drugs to be a criminal act plainly implies that the person freely chose to use those drugs and could reasonably have decided otherwise.

The more recent view sees addiction as a disease and addicts as individuals in need of treatment. This view first gained momentum in the United States with the repeal of alcohol prohibition in 1933. During the Prohibition era, most U.S. public education efforts taught that alcohol was a drug so hazardous that no one could drink it safely and in moderation. Making alcohol once again legally and widely available thus posed a conundrum in public and professional opinion: why were we unleashing this pernicious drug on the public? This dissonance was resolved by concluding that only certain people (alcoholics) were at risk and incapable of using alcohol in moderation, by virtue of a disease that rendered them different from normal individuals. For these unfortunate people, abstinence was the answer, whereas the rest of humanity could drink with impunity. This simplistic disease model has since given way to a more sophisticated neurobiological understanding of how the use of certain drugs can become a self-perpetuating cycle.

If there is a point on which these two models agree, it is that motivation is a central factor in addiction. Within a volitional view, the user needs to be sufficiently motivated to say no to drugs. Such motivation might be enhanced by persuasion, education, punishment, confrontation, reinforcement of nonuse, or appealing to the person's higher values. In a neurobiological view, it is precisely the motivational systems of the brain that are hijacked. The most addictive drugs are those that directly stimulate positive reinforcement and pain relief channels of the central nervous system, sending the message, "Do that again!" Animal models of learning and neuroadaptation are sufficient to explain how human beings can fall into addiction (Logan, 1993). What we lack is an adequate animal model to explain the kind of recovery that occurs in Alcoholics Anonymous (AA) and treatment.

In both volitional and neurobiological views there is also the potential for a gradual weakening of self-control over time. From a volitional perspective, the person becomes a victim of habit. The human capacity for self-control fatigues, enhancing susceptibility to temptation. Like abstaining, giving in to temptation once makes it easier to do it the next time, and sometimes it is the very effort to restrain oneself that increases the likelihood of relapse. Similarly, neuroadaptation involves biological changes in response to drug use that increase the likelihood of repetition and escalation, gradually undermining the person's capacity for volitional control.

Human will is seldom completely free, though few would maintain that choice plays no role whatsoever in human behavior. One possibility is to think of choice as accounting for a fluctuating percentage of the variation in human action. Some behaviors are more readily susceptible to willful control than are others—e.g., watching television versus slowing one's heart rate—and there are individual differences in overall capacity for volitional control—e.g., impulsivity and attention deficit / hyperactivity disorders. Even for the same behavior in the same individual, capacity for self-control varies over time depending on a host of factors, such as fatigue, mood, and salience of temptation. Subjectively, the addictive behaviors are those that more people have more trouble regulating more of the time. Nevertheless, the reality of choice and responsibility for one's behavior remains.

A volitional, or choice, perspective helps make sense of some puzzling findings in addiction treatment and recovery (Vuchinich and Heather, 2003). One of these is that the vast majority of people who recover from addictions—be it addiction to tobacco (nicotine), alcohol, or illicit drugs—do so on their own without formal treatment. When asked how they did it, many say "I just decided" or recall a particular turning point at which things changed. Another puzzling finding is responsiveness to brief intervention. Dozens of randomized trials show that people with alcohol use disorders are significantly more likely to reduce or stop their drinking if given brief advice or counseling (usually a session or two) than if nothing is done. Often the effect of such brief counseling is just as large as that for more extensive treatment. Then there is the finding that most of the reduction in substance use that follows treatment tends to occur during the first few sessions and sometimes even before the person begins treatment. Motivational interviewing (MI) was specifically designed to help tip the decisional balance regarding substance use and increase readiness for change by evoking the individual's own motivations. Like other brief interventions, MI has been found to trigger change in substance use, and a session or two of MI at the beginning of a longer course of treatment can substantially improve outcomes (Hettema et al., 2005). All of this suggests that people with substance use disorders reach a decision to turn the corner.

This choice perspective is not incompatible with neurobiological, or disease, views of addiction. Although neurobiological models clarify the ways in which self-control is undermined, ultimately it is the individual who has the choice and responsibility of recovery. Few would promise that a medication, therapy, or AA will succeed for the person without his or her active involvement. AA members make the decision to turn their will over to a higher power, choose not to drink one day at a time, and observe that "it works if you work it." Under laboratory conditions, even severely addicted individuals can and do make choices about using available drugs in response to environmental contingencies. Apart from closely supervised incarceration, it is the individual who must ultimately work out whether and how to live in a community unencumbered by drug use.

Both volitional choice and neurobiological perspectives point to motivational factors as central to addictions and recovery. This suggests that efforts to prevent, reduce, and treat addictions could be guided by research findings about human motivation and could focus on approaches that help people choose life unimpaired by substance use (or addictive behaviors more generally). Outcome research on what actually works in prevention and treatment is consistent with this perspective. As Surgeon General Koop observes in this volume, measures that limit the availability and increase the price of addictive substances like alcohol and tobacco substantially diminish their use. The methods found to be most effective in treating substance use disorders also tend to target motivational factors (Miller et al., 2003; Miller and Carroll, 2006). Brief interventions and MI emphasize the person's freedom of choice and encourage change in substance use, without providing much specific guidance in how to do so. Two other evidence-based treatment methods—the community reinforcement approach (Meyers and Smith, 1995) and contingency management (Higgins and Petry, 1999) specifically focus on increasing positive reinforcement and social support for sobriety, making a drug-free life too good to abandon. Effective medications provide temporary insurance against impulsive use (e.g., disulfiram for alcohol, naltrexone for heroin), reduced incentive for use (e.g., naltrexone for alcohol, buprenorphine for heroin), and/or a more stable source of drug reinforcement (e.g., methadone, nicotine patch). A majority of drug users who refuse to get help can be engaged in treatment by teaching their loved ones how to motivate change.

Finally, it is important to emphasize that the volitional and neurobiological perspectives on addiction do not correspond to harsh versus compassionate treatment of the afflicted, respectively. Punishment is notoriously ineffective in suppressing well-established alcohol, tobacco, or other drug use, particularly (though not only) when the person can escape the negative consequences. Research has shown that confrontational counseling approaches are abysmally ineffective (Miller et al., 2003). Coercive attempts to take away the person's choice and responsibility or to invoke shame ultimately fail to change behavior. There is every reason to treat the victims of substance use disorders with empathy and compassion, not only because it is the humane thing to do but also because it is effective in motivating change.

So, yes, addiction has much to do with self-control. The impairment of self-control is a subjective hallmark of addictions, for which there is ample neurobiological evidence. Some individuals who come to the attention of treatment, correctional, health, and social service systems show generalized difficulties in self-regulation. Others simply were ensnared in the escalating cycle of neuroadaptation. Whatever the etiology, it is our task to treat people with dignity, autonomy, and compassion, providing whatever help we can to tip their decisional balance in the direction of life instead of destruction.

REFERENCES

Hettema, J., Steele, J., and Miller, W. R. 2005. Motivational interviewing. *Annual Review of Clinical Psychology* 1:91–111.

Higgins, S.T., and Petry, N.M. 1999. Contingency management: incentives for sobriety. *Alcohol Research and Health* 23:122–27.

Logan, F.A. 1993. Animal learning and motivation and addictive drugs. *Psychological Reports* 73:291–306.

Meyers, R. J., and Smith, J. E. 1995. *Clinical Guide to Alcohol Treatment: The Community Reinforcement Approach*. New York: Guilford Press.

Miller, W. R., and Carroll, K. M., eds. 2006. *Rethinking Substance Abuse: What the Science Shows, and What We Should Do about It*. New York: Guilford Press.

Miller, W. R., Wilbourne, P. L., and Hettema, J. E. 2003. What works? A summary of alcohol treatment outcome research. In: R. K. Hester and W. R. Miller, eds., *Handbook of Alcoholism Treatment Approaches: Effective Alternatives*, 3rd ed. Boston: Allyn & Bacon.

Vuchinich, R. E., and Heather, N., eds. 2003. *Choice, Behavioral Economics and Addiction*. New York: Pergamon Press.

2

The P.R.I.M.E. Theory of Motivation as a Possible Foundation for the Treatment of Addiction

ROBERT WEST, PH.D., B.SC.

We would, ideally, like to find effective "cures" for addictions as we have for some cancers. With a cure, the addict's disordered motivational system would be "restored to health" and the addictive behavior would no longer have a dominant place in his or her motivational hierarchy. Failing that, we strive to find effective therapies that suppress addictive disorders, like therapies we currently have for HIV infection, and, if we cannot achieve that, we search for ways of "managing" addictions so that we limit the damage they cause, perhaps in the way we manage asthma.

Our success at doing any of these things depends on our understanding of what is wrong with the addict. At present we have some idea (for a comprehensive review of theories, see West, [2006]). In a susceptible individual, particular behaviors (mostly drug-taking behaviors) get out of control because they change the individual's central nervous system (CNS) and/or social and physical environment to increase the motivation to seek out and engage in the activity. This can be because an artificial "drive" is created, abstinence becomes unpleasant, the behavior is rewarding, the rewards and punishments associated with the behavior establish powerful habits of thought, feeling, or action, or the ability or will to resist the motivation to engage in the behavior becomes diminished.

We can go beyond this and say what changes take place in the CNS, what it is about the behaviors that is rewarding, what underpins the unpleasant effects of abstinence, how the social environment changes to promote deepening dependence, and how it is that our propensity to exercise self-control is weakened. We have many plausible hypotheses at varying levels of analysis, from the biochemical to the sociological.

Where has this understanding gotten us so far? We do not yet seem to have any kind of cure for heroin addiction, but with long-term opiate substitution treatments (primarily methadone and buprenorphine) we can often keep it at bay, and with counseling and needle-exchange programs we can sometimes reduce problematic behaviors (Lingford-Hughes et al., 2004). For cocaine addiction, we have no demonstrated cure, and no therapy to keep it at bay, but counseling may help reduce problematic use (Lingford-Hughes et al., 2004). The same is probably true for amphetamine addiction. For alcohol addiction, it is arguable that some people are cured by a combination of medication and counseling, but more commonly it is kept at bay so that even alcoholics who are "dry" are susceptible to relapse (Lingford-Hughes et al., 2004). It looks as though nicotine addiction can be cured in perhaps 5 percent of cases by a course of medication, such as nicotine-replacement therapy, and in perhaps 10 percent by a combination of medication and what is termed "behavioral support" (Lingford-Hughes et al., 2004). There is little experience of trying to treat this addiction long term or to offer interventions to mitigate the harm. For gambling addiction, medications that improve or stabilize mood or control impulsiveness and psychological treatments have shown promise, at least in managing the disorder (Toneatto and Millar, 2004).

Conceptualizing Addiction

We may be able to do better than this. It is worth examining in more detail the phenomenon with which we are attempting to deal. Strangely, there does not seem to be a strong consensus concerning what the phenomenon is. Some researchers regard it as primarily a problem of making maladaptive choices (Skog, 2000), some regard it as a problem of biases in the way people implicitly think about the costs and benefits of the activities (Brown et al., 1987), some focus on powerful feelings of compulsion that addicts experience (Jellinek, 1960), others argue that there is some kind of deficit in the mechanism we use to inhibit responses (Lubman et al., 2004), still others focus on the notion of "habit" (O'Brien et al., 1992), and yet others place emphasis on how the addict places himself or herself in the social environment (Kearney and O'Sullivan, 2003). For some researchers and clinicians, addiction and dependence mean the same thing, while others distinguish between physical dependence and psychological addiction. And I have recently argued for a distinction between addiction (a reward-seeking behavior that has gotten out of control) and the range of different "dependence syndromes" that are associated with different drugs (e.g., tolerance, withdrawal symptoms, narrowing of repertoire, etc. [West, 2006]).

It is unlikely that a consensus will emerge because there is no objective way of deciding the issue. There is no pathogen as there is with, say, malaria, and no obvious structural abnormality as there is with a bone fracture. We can, however, build up a picture of the motivational system and the ways in which behavior patterns that we call "addiction" and others that are "addiction-like" emerge. In doing so, perhaps we can gain some new insights that will help us understand the limitations of the treatments we are currently using and ways in which we might improve things for the future.

Plans-Responses-Impulses-Motives-Evaluation: The P.R.I.M.E. Theory of Motivation

A great deal is known about human motivation, but, surprisingly, it has not until now been put together into a synthetic theory. Thus, there is a wealth of ideas on judgment and decision making, emotions, drives, habits, reflexes, and so on, but they have not been integrated into a model of the motivational system as a whole. I have attempted to draft such an integration (West, 2006). The result is necessarily complex, but there are five unifying themes: the structure of the motivational system; focus on the moment; neural plasticity; identity, self-awareness, and self-control; and the unstable mind.

Theme 1: The Structure of the Motivational System

The first theme is a statement about the overall structure of the "motivational system." It is claimed that this system operates at five levels of complexity as shown in Figure 2.1. At the lowest level are the responses themselves (starting, stopping, or modifying actions). At the next level are impulses and inhibitory forces. These are forces that

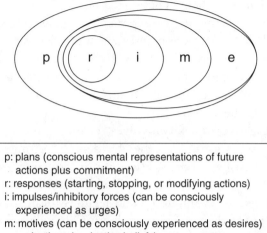

p: plans (conscious mental representations of future
   actions plus commitment)
r: responses (starting, stopping, or modifying actions)
i: impulses/inhibitory forces (can be consciously
   experienced as urges)
m: motives (can be consciously experienced as desires)
e: evaluations (evaluative beliefs)

Figure 2.1. The structure of the motivational system. Responses are generated directly by the internal and external environment, as in reflexes, and by impulses and inhibitory forces. They are influenced directly by the internal and external environment and often also by motives, which are often experienced as feelings of desire or want; these experiences, in turn, are influenced directly but sometimes by evaluations, which are beliefs about what is good or bad, right or wrong, useful or harmful. We are sometimes motivated to form plans, which are mental representations of actions together with some level of intention and starting conditions. Those plans may then later influence motives or evaluations. The external environment is filtered through the internal environment. Evaluations can influence responses only through motives, which can influence responses only through impulses. This structure gives an inherent advantage to events that directly generate impulses over, for example, those that influence beliefs about what is harmful.

impel and restrain specific actions and are the final common pathway through which all higher-order motivational elements operate. Environmental events, emotional states, and internal drives can generate impulses directly (e.g., frustration leading to the impulse to act aggressively, hunger leading to the impulse to eat). If impulses are uncontested we do not experience any feelings associated with them, but if they are held back for any reason we experience them as "urges."

Impulses "push" our behavior. The higher levels of motivation "pull" behavior in the sense that they are future-oriented. First, there are what may be called "motives." These are mental representations of objects, events, and so forth, together with a degree of attraction or repulsion attached to them. These need not be brought to conscious awareness, but when they are we experience them as feelings of "want," "desire," or "need." Attraction and repulsion arise out of anticipated feelings of contentment and distress. If we have conflicting motives, the one that is strongest at the time will create the impulse to action. That impulse will then compete with any other impulses present at the time to generate the action.

The next level of complexity involves "evaluations." These are propositional representations about the world as it is or might be that involve some sense of good or bad (useful or detrimental, morally right or wrong, etc.). This theory draws a fundamental distinction between motivational beliefs (evaluations) and feelings (desires and urges). A strong claim of the theory is that evaluations have no direct effect on our actions. They must work through motives and then impulses. The hierarchy of levels of motivation confers a natural advantage on impulses over desires and desires over evaluations in the control of our moment-to-moment behavior.

The fifth and final level of complexity in the structure of motivations is the "plan." Humans are capable of forming mental representations of actions together with a set of more or less well-defined "starting conditions" and a degree of "commitment" to them. This allows for considerably more flexibility of action than would otherwise be possible. Desires that cannot be fulfilled at present because of other priorities or practicalities can be met at a future date. We can also construct plans in anticipation of future events that will deliver opportunities or threats. The main problem with plans is that they have to be remembered in order to generate the evaluations and motives necessary to control our actions.

Theme 2: The Focus on the Moment

The second unifying theme is the focus on the "moment." Our actions at any one time can only be influenced by forces operating at that time. Urges, desires, plans, and evaluations can affect behavior only at the time they are active. When they are not active, all that exists is the structural configuration of synapses in the CNS that give them the potential to be generated. This self-evident thesis is largely overlooked in theories of motivation that postulate concepts such as "cognition," "attitude," and "intention" as stable entities of uncertain epistemological status. The focus in the P.R.I.M.E. theory is on the dynamic and fluid nature of motivation and behavior. Such consistencies as exist in the way we respond to events arise from the fact that the same CNS structural configuration is being acted on by the same inputs to regenerate the same motives.

This provides a natural basis for explaining why, despite every "intention" to change the way one responds to a situation, one often finds oneself doing the same thing one did before. It also highlights the critical importance of motivation to avoid or escape from unpleasant thoughts as well as unpleasant experiences: not thinking about things is one of our most widely used coping strategies.

Theme 3: Neural Plasticity

The third unifying theme concerns the ways in which the motivational system is altered in the short, medium, and long term by experience. The theory identifies three types of plasticity: habituation/sensitization, in which merely repeating a stimulus makes it less or more attractive or repellent; explicit memory, in which experiences and ideas can be regenerated in a more or less similar form given appropriate cues; and associative learning, which includes classical conditioning (stimulus-stimulus associations) and instrumental conditioning (stimulus-response-reinforcement associations). Associative learning results in causal connections between patterns of activity in the motivational system (including experiences, feelings, responses) becoming more "habitual" (i.e., rapid) and involving less attention.

Theme 4: Identity, Self-Awareness, and Self-Control

The fourth unifying theme is the critical importance of "identity" and "self-awareness" and the role that these have in "self-control." We are obviously capable of forming mental representations of ourselves and equally obviously those mental representations have a special significance. In keeping with the focus on the moment, we need to be attentive to the fact that those mental representations exist only when they are generated and the form they take depends partly on the structural configuration of our CNS and partly on whatever else is going on in our heads at the time. Like any mental representation, they can be coherent and detailed or incoherent and vague, they can be multifaceted or simple, and they can focus on one feature at one time and other features at other times.

One important influence that our self-concepts have on our motivation stems from evaluation of ourselves. This influences the contentment or distress we feel when we think about ourselves, and how much we like or dislike ourselves. This has widespread ramifications that affect all self-conscious behavior.

Self-awareness is a prerequisite for self-control. According to the P.R.I.M.E. theory, self-control consists of the operation of evaluations and motives that stem from self-awareness. To exercise self-control to stop myself doing something, I must be aware of myself and my desires must include myself in that mental representation. Un-self-conscious inhibition of a response (for example, because of a distracting or shock stimulus) would not count. Self-control is therefore based on a desire or evaluation concerning oneself (e.g., I want to be a nonsmoker).

This has some important and unobvious implications. For ex-

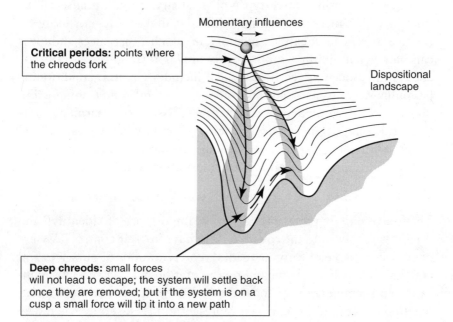

Figure 2.2. An example of Waddington's epigenetic landscape. The state of a system at a given time is represented by the position of a ball in the landscape. The landscape itself unfolds and represents potential paths down which systems may develop while environmental forces move the ball laterally in that landscape. Small forces at critical moments can send the system down an ever-deepening valley. Once in that valley, large and/or sustained forces are needed to move it into a different one.

ample, if thinking about myself is distressing, I will be less inclined to entertain self-awareness and hence less likely to exercise self-control.

Under the theory, self-control requires mental effort, which in turn requires reserves of mental energy. Like physical energy this becomes depleted through use.

Theme 5: The Unstable Mind

The fifth unifying theme is application of "chaos theory" to the motivational system. Human motivation is much more like a weather system than it is like domestic plumbing. Motivation is inherently unstable and kept more or less in check by constant balancing input. It is continually inclined to head off down a new path unless it is kept on course. Chaos theory is a mathematical system for explaining, among other things, how systems can at one time appear to be deeply entrenched in a particular pattern of activity but suddenly switch to another. It explains how the tiniest of influences at a critical time can send the system down an ever-deepening rut. It deals with predicting over a period of time what is unpredictable at any given moment in time.

The single most useful concept for our purposes is Waddington's visual model of the "epigenetic landscape" (originally developed to model embryological development [Waddington 1977]). Waddington's image suggests a way of modeling how environmental influences interact with the structure of the motivational system to generate behaviors (Figure 2.2).

What P.R.I.M.E. Theory Means for Addiction

Addiction metastasizes into the entire motivational system. Because of the causal links between different elements in the motivational system, there will be many cases (probably the large majority) in which the distortion in priorities involves multiple levels. Strong habits are supported by and support powerful desires, and they are justified by firmly held beliefs. In a "mature" addiction it will be rare that a single rogue element in the system is responsible for the addictive pattern of behavior even though it may have been necessary for its initiation.

It is unhelpful to categorize addicts in terms of "stage of change." Motivation to attempt to "give up" or "control" an addictive behavior pattern is fluid and highly situationally determined. Even small triggers can lead to sudden conversion-like transformations of the system, which then lead to lasting change. To label individuals in terms of their "stage of change" (Prochaska et al., 1992) is fundamentally to misrepresent the process of motivation to change addictive behaviors (West, 2005).

Clinical assessment of addicts can usefully be structured around the five themes of P.R.I.M.E. theory. The purpose of clinical assessment is to provide a basis for prognosis and treatment. The therapist needs to be aware of the prospects for the addict of cure, suppression, or management of the condition. Based on the five themes outlined above, assessment should (1) encompass all relevant levels of motivation to gain an understanding of how far the distortions in the motivational system have become manifest in impulses, desires, evaluations, and plans; (2) delineate the pattern of environmental triggers acting on the addict to determine the momentary environmental influences that pose a threat to change; (3) determine the results of neural plasticity in terms of acquired habits, drives, and so forth to ascertain the importance of implicit and explicit expectancies, habits, and acquired drives in maintaining the behavior; (4) establish the involvement of identity to assess the barriers to exercise self-control and how far embedded the addiction is in the addict's/patient's self-concept; and (5) evaluate the susceptibility of the addict to possible intervention strategies to determine what are the realistic prospects for shifting the state of the motivational system to a new pathway.

The treatment program needs to involve multiple components targeted at all the modifiable distortions in the motivational system. Because addiction will usually involve distortions across the entire system, the treatment program needs to address all elements that can be affected, for as long as is necessary either to achieve a cure or to suppress the addiction. In most cases, a cure is probably unrealistic because habits, acquired drives, expectancies, and sense of identity are too deeply established and because whatever personal and environmental characteristics made the individual susceptible to the development of addiction usually remain in place.

The focus needs to be on identifying the most appropriate targets for change, bearing in mind resources and ethical and practical limitations. Both medication and psychological techniques should be considered. Medications might be used to reduce acquired drive states, discomfort associated with abstinence, and emotional states that undermine self-control, as well as mitigate generalized impulse control problems and block selectively the reward provided by the activity. Psychological techniques can be used to try to engender a radical change in identity—a kind of conversion experience leading to a fundamental change in the evaluations underpinning the addiction—and engender new habits of thought, feeling, and behavior. A third possibility is to reshape the addict's social and physical environment as far as possible to minimize the immediate triggers for the behavior, increase rewards for exercising control and disincentives for the addictive behavior, and provide distractions.

Many current approaches, such as nicotine replacement therapy and motivational interviewing, each address some of these targets. P.R.I.M.E. theory provides a principled basis for combining different treatment elements to achieve maximum effect and, where resources are limited, for choosing which target elements of the motivational system to focus on in which cases.

Making New Men and Women

In all this, we need to recognize that except in rare cases we are not carrying out the psychological equivalent of surgically removing a tumor from an otherwise healthy body. We are seeking to reshape the addict's motivational system—to change the addict as a person. In some cases this may go to the root of his or her being. Perhaps we should hope that our techniques for doing this never become too successful because in the wrong hands . . .

REFERENCES

Brown, S. A., Christiansen, B. A., and Goldman, M. S. 1987. The Alcohol Expectancy Questionnaire: an instrument for the assessment of adolescent and adult alcohol expectancies. *Journal of Studies on Alcohol* 48:483–91.

Jellinek, E. M. 1960. *The Disease Concept of Alcoholism.* New Brunswick, N.J.: Hillhouse Press.

Kearney, M. H., and O'Sullivan, J. 2003. Identity shifts as turning points in health behavior change. *Western Journal of Nursing Research* 25: 134–52.

Lingford-Hughes, A. R., Welch, S., and Nutt, D. J. 2004. Evidence-based guidelines for the pharmacological management of substance misuse, addiction and comorbidity: recommendations from the British Association for Psychopharmacology. *Journal of Psychopharmacology* 18:293–335.

Lubman, D. I., Yucel, M., and Pantelis, C. 2004. Addiction, a condition of compulsive behavior? Neuroimaging and neuropsychological evidence of inhibitory dysregulation. *Addiction* 99:1491–502.

O'Brien, C. P., Childress, A. R., McLellan, A. T., and Ehrman, R. 1992. A learning model of addiction. *Research Publications—Association for Research in Nervous and Mental Disease* 70:157–77.

Prochaska, J. O., DiClemente, C. C., and Norcross, J. C. 1992. In search of how people change: applications to addictive behaviors. *American Psychologist* 47:1102–14.

Skog, O. J. 2000. Addicts' choice. *Addiction* 95:1309–14.

Toneatto, T., and Millar, G. 2004. Assessing and treating problem gambling: empirical status and promising trends. *Canadian Journal of Psychiatry* 49:517–25.

Waddington, C. 1997. *Tools for Thought: How to Understand and Apply the Latest Scientific Techniques of Problem Solving.* New York: Basic Books.

West, R. 2005. Time for a change: putting the Transtheoretical (Stages of Change) Model to rest. *Addiction* 100:1036–39.

West, R. 2006. *Theory of Addiction.* Oxford, England: Blackwell's.

3

A Future for the Prevention and Treatment of Drug Abuse
Applications of Computer-Based Interactive Technology

WARREN K. BICKEL, PH.D., AND
LISA A. MARSCH, PH.D.

A positive, substantive impact on the problems of substance use disorders in the United States requires a reassessment and reorganization of how we prevent and treat drug abuse. Despite important scientific advances in preventing and treating drug abuse and dependence, the current prevention and treatment system faces numerous, serious challenges, including high demand, limited availability of services, difficulty recruiting and retaining providers of service, limited financing for services, and slow adoption of evidence-based innovations (Bickel and McLellan, 1996; McLellan et al., 2003). Increases in substance use disorders in rural communities present additional important challenges with respect to access, availability, and cost-effectiveness of prevention and treatment.

Unfortunately, for the foreseeable future, the likelihood of substantial increases in financial support for enhancements in prevention and treatment services is low. If we wish to increase and improve services, the only viable alternative is to consider new approaches. These new approaches must be not only effective and evidence-based but also substantially less costly than expanding the number of service providers and training them to deliver the latest evidence-based approaches.

New information technologies offer just such an opportunity. Although information technology is bringing profound changes to our society in many areas, it is just beginning to be employed in the field of drug abuse prevention and treatment. It has the potential, however, to address many of the challenges associated with the current delivery of services for substance use disorders. In light of the potential benefits of innovative use of this technology and its potential to play a central role in the future of the field, we provide a brief overview of computer-based interactive technology, a synopsis of research conducted to date related to the application of computer technology to substance use disorders, and a vision of the future for drug abuse prevention and treatment.

Overview of Computer-Based Interactive Technology

Computer-based interactive technologies refer to "computer-based media that enable users to access information and services of interest, control how the information is presented, and respond to information and messages in a mediated environment (e.g., answer questions, send a message, take an action in a game, receive feedback, or make a response to previous actions)" (Street and Rimal, 1997, p. 2). Two central features of this technology are interactivity and modularity (Street and Rimal, 1997). "Interactivity" refers to the responsiveness of the program to the behavior of the user and to the ability of the user to modify or control the presentation of material (Rafaeli, 1988; Steuer, 1992). "Modularity" refers to program design that enables the user to access different portions of a program and to move from one portion to another easily (Dede and Fontana, 1995; Street and Rimal, 1997). Types of computer-based interactive technology that have been employed to deliver therapy include desktop computers (Selmi et al., 1990), e-mail (Murphy and Mitchell, 1998), hand-held devices (Newman et al., 1997b), telephone-accessed computer systems (Osgood-Hynes et al, 1998), video-disc training (Thorkildsen et al., 1979), virtual reality systems (North et al., 1997), and web-based interventions (Wantland et al., 2004). The disorders for which computers have been employed to provide treatment or promote health behaviors include Alzheimer disease (Brennan et al., 1995), arthritis (Wetstone et al., 1985), asthma (Rubin et al., 1986), anxiety (Newman et al., 1997b), depression (Selmi et al., 1990), diabetes (Wise et al., 1986), heart disease (Lyons et al., 1982), HIV (Gustafson et al., 1994), and hypertension (Ben-Said et al., 1994).

Computerized treatments for psychiatric disorders have been most widely developed and used for anxiety and depressive disorders (Buglione et al., 1990; Selmi et al., 1990; Newman et al., 1996, 1997b; for a review, see Newman et al. [1997a]). The development of computer-based interventions for the treatment of these disorders may, in part, be a result of the manuals developed for cognitive-behavioral treatments of these disorders—that is, manual-driven treatments that specify the use of certain sequences of procedures may be readily adapted for computer-based interventions (Selmi et al., 1990). The increasing number of manual-driven therapies in drug abuse, supports the value of considering the development of computer based treatments. It is interesting, and most important for the considerations of this chapter, that comparisons of computer-delivered and therapist-delivered treatments in anxiety and depressive disorders have generally reported comparable outcomes (Carr et al., 1988; Ghosh et al., 1988; Buglione et al., 1990).

Applications of Computer-Based Interactive Technology to Substance Abuse

The use of computers in substance abuse prevention and treatment is a small but growing research area. To the best of our knowledge, only four controlled studies have been published that examine the efficacy of interactive, computer-delivered interventions focused on prevention (one study) and treatment (three studies) of substance use disorders.

The prevention study evaluated a computer-assisted, school-based substance abuse prevention program for middle school–aged adolescents called "HeadOn: Substance Abuse Prevention for Grades 6–8" (Marsch et al., 2007). This self-guided program was designed to deliver evidence-based education about effective drug abuse prevention to youth in order to promote the learning of key skills and information. HeadOn was found to promote significantly higher levels of accuracy in objective knowledge about drug abuse prevention than the demonstrably effective Life Skills Training Program with which it was compared. In addition, participants in the HeadOn and Life Skills groups generally achieved comparable, positive outcomes after completing their substance abuse prevention intervention on a wide variety of measures, including self-reported rates of substance use, intentions to use substances, attitudes toward substances, beliefs about prevalence of substance use among both their peers and adults, and likelihood of refusing a drug offer. Moreover, HeadOn proved to be cost-effective relative to Life Skills for middle school youth in a school-based setting: analysis showed that costs for HeadOn were slightly more than half those of Life Skills.

The first treatment study randomly assigned 40 heavy drinkers to receive a computerized version of a behavioral self-control training program either immediately after pretreatment assessment or after a ten-week waiting period (Hester and Delaney, 1997). Patients who received the computer-based intervention significantly reduced their drinking (average 13.8–14.5 drinks per week) as compared both to their pretreatment levels (35.2 drinks per week) and to patients in the delayed treatment group (34.3 drinks per week). Moreover, after receiving the intervention, the delayed treatment group significantly reduced their drinking from an average of 34 drinks per week to 20.8 drinks per week. A 12-month follow-up demonstrated that patients maintained the treatment gains.

The second treatment study provided an interactive behavioral smoking cessation program on the CompuServe computer network (Schneider et al., 1990). The 1,158 participants were randomly dispersed among four treatment groups in a two-by-two design: one of two intervention groups receiving the full computer-based smoking-cessation program, one with and one without a stop smoking online forum, or to one of two control groups receiving a (sham) computer program with and without the online forum. Overall, use of these resources was poor, though abstinence rates were significantly better at one-and three-month follow-ups for individuals who received the full program than for those who received the control treatment, regardless of whether they had access to the online forum. At the six-month follow-up, there was no difference among the groups, though data suggested slightly better rates of abstinence for those who received the full program (e.g., regardless of access to the online forum).

The third treatment study compared computer-delivered to therapist-delivered HIV/AIDS education among opioid-dependent, injection drug-users (IDUs) receiving buprenorphine treatment (Marsch and Bickel, 2004). Thirty participants were randomly assigned to receive HIV/AIDS education delivered either by a computer or by counselors. Patients who received computer-based instruction learned significantly more information than did counselor-educated participants and retained significantly more of that information at a three-month follow-up. In addition, participants in the computer-based training condition liked the teaching medium significantly better than those in the therapist-delivered program. It is important to note that significantly more patients who received the computer-based training answered affirmatively when asked whether they would like to receive more information about AIDS, including HIV/AIDS pamphlets and information on being tested for HIV. Individuals in both conditions exhibited comparable and significant reductions in HIV risk behavior. This study demonstrated that computer-based HIV/AIDS education might provide a systematic and effective intervention that is attractive to IDUs and that may be cost-effective.

If demonstrated to be effective, therapeutic applications of computer-based interactive technology in the treatment of substance use disorders may provide at least seven advantages over the current treatment system of in-person care, including: (1) increased access to prevention and treatment for individuals with substance use disorders, (2) speedier dissemination of innovative psychological prevention and treatment programs within the professional community, (3) greater consistency in the delivery of the intervention, (4) more user friendly or less threatening (particularly when addressing sensitive issues such as HIV risk behavior), (5) reduced cost to deliver treatment or prevention programs, (6) enhanced feasibility of long-term therapeutic activities, and (7) increased opportunities for patient self-review of necessary skills training and completion therapeutic tasks.

Envisioning the Future of Drug Abuse Prevention and Treatment

If additional study of computer-based interactive technology continues to demonstrate its effectiveness and cost-effectiveness, it could permit us to extend, expand, and reorganize our system for providing prevention and treatment services. Prevention service in the twenty-first century might include access to prevention software throughout the educational experience from elementary school through college, enabling school personnel to focus greater efforts on youth who are at considerably greater risk for drug use or perhaps have started use. Versions of these programs could be devised so that children and their parents could work on aspects of the program together, thereby facilitating discussion and interaction as they address this important matter.

Inclusion of computer-based interventions as part of treatment in the twenty-first century may help expand treatment. First, computer-delivered therapies could widely extend the availability of treatment via the Internet. Individuals seeking treatment could sign up for treatment remotely and participate from their homes or any place providing access to the Internet (e.g., libraries, community centers). Such a treatment package could also easily support a hybrid model in which therapists discuss the results of the computer treatment and assessment with the patient. Such a hybrid model could be a standard aspect of treatment or alternatively could be reserved for those individuals who do not make sufficient progress with the computer application. By providing some aspects of therapeutic interventions via computer, therapists may be better able to focus on providing those aspects of therapy that they are uniquely trained to address.

Another important potential application of this method of delivering care is what we will refer to as continuity of care. In most contemporary treatments, individuals often can receive extensive (and often expensive) treatment when there is an acute exacerbation in their substance abuse. Once the treatment episode is concluded, there often is little or no ongoing, chronic care. Indeed, chronic care would be fiscally challenging to consider. With computerized therapy, however, such care could be provided with minimal cost and may aid in delaying or preventing relapse.

The future of prevention and treatment efforts must not only be in the development of effective prevention and treatment approaches but also address how to deliver them so that they have the broadest reach and greatest opportunity to positively affect the drug use problems facing our country. The use of computer-based interactive technologies is an important positive, cost-effective step that is expanding access to evidence-based approaches.

ACKNOWLEDGMENTS

Preparation of this chapter was supported by grant R01 DA 12997 from the National Institute on Drug Abuse. Some portions of this chapter were adapted from Bickel, Marsch, Buchhalter, and Badger (under review). The authors appreciate the comments of Benjamin Kowal on an earlier version of this chapter.

REFERENCES

Ben-Said, M., Consoli, S., and Jean, J. 1994. A comparative study between a computer-aided education (ISIS) and habitual education techniques for hypertensive patients. *Proceedings of the Annual Symposium on Computer Applications in Medical Care* 10–14.

Bickel, W. K., and McLellan, A. T. 1996. Can management by outcome invigorate substance abuse treatment? *American Journal on Addictions* 5:281–91.

Brennan, P. F., Moore, S. M., and Smyth, K. A. 1995. The effects of a special computer network on caregivers of persons with Alzheimer's disease. *Nursing Research* 44:166–72.

Buglione, S. A., Devito, A. J., and Mulloy, J. M. 1990. Traditional group therapy and computer-administered treatment for test anxiety. *Anxiety Research* 3:33–39.

Carr, A. C., Ghosh, A., and Marks, I. M. 1988. Computer-supervised exposure treatment for phobias. *Canadian Journal of Psychiatry* 33:112–17.

Dede, C., and Fontana, L. 1995. Transforming health education via new media. In L. M. Harris, ed., *Health and the New Media: Technologies Transforming Personal and Public Health*. Hillsdale, N.J.: Erlbaum.

Ghosh, A., Marks, I. M., Carr, A. C. 1988. Therapist contact and outcome of self-exposure treatment for phobias: a controlled study. *British Journal of Psychiatry* 152:234–38.

Gustafson, D. H., Hawkins, R. P., Boberg, E. W., Bricker, E., Pingree, S., and Chan, C. 1994. The use and impact of a computer-based support system for people living with AIDS and HIV infection. *Proceedings of the Annual Symposium on Computer Applications in Medical Care* 604–8.

Hester, R. K., and Delaney, H. D. 1997. Behavioral self-control program for Windows: results of a controlled clinical trial. *Journal of Consulting and Clinical Psychology* 65:685–93.

Lyons, C., Krasnowski, J., Greenstein, A., Maloney, D., and Tatarczuk, J. 1982. Interactive computerized patient education. *Heart and Lung* 11:340–41.

Marsch, L. A., and Bickel, W. K. 2004. The efficacy of computer-based HIV/AIDS education for injection drug users. *American Journal of Health Behavior* 28:316–27.

Marsch, L. A., Bickel, W. K., and Badger, G. J. 2007. Applying computer technology to substance abuse prevention science. *Journal of Child and Adolescent Substance Abuse* 16:69–94.

Murphy, L. J., and Mitchell, D. L. 1998. When writing helps to heal: e-mail as therapy. *British Journal of Guidance and Counseling* 26:21–32.

McLellan, A. T., Carise, D., and Kleber, H. D. 2003. Can the national addiction treatment infrastructure support the public's demand for quality care? *Journal of Substance Abuse Treatment* 25:117–21.

Newman, M. G., Kenardy, J., Herman, S., and Taylor, C. B. 1996. The use of hand-held computers as an adjunct to cognitive-behavior therapy. *Computers in Human Behavior* 12:135–43.

Newman, M. G., Consoli, A., and Taylor, C. B. 1997a. Computers in the assessment and cognitive behavior treatment of clinical disorders: anxiety as the case in point. *Behavior Therapy* 28:211–35.

Newman, M. G., Kenardy, J., Herman, S., and Taylor, C. B. 1997b. Comparison of cognitive-behavioral treatment of panic disorder with computer assisted brief cognitive behavioral treatment. *Journal of Consulting and Clinical Psychology* 65:178–83.

North, M. M., North, S. M., and Coble, J. R. 1997. *Virtual Reality Therapy: An Innovative Paradigm*. Colorado Springs, Colo.: IPI Press.

Osgood-Hynes, D. J., Greist, J. H., Marks, I. M., Baer, L., Heneman, S. W., Wenzel, K. W., Manzo, P. A., Parkins, J. R., Spierings, C. J., Dottl, S. L., and Vitse, H. M. 1998. Self-administered psychotherapy for depression using a telephone-accessed computer system plus booklets: an open U.S.-U.K. study. *Journal of Clinical Psychiatry* 59:358–65.

Rafaeli, S. 1988. Interactivity: from new media to communication. *Sage Annual Review of Communication Research: Advancing Communication Science* 16:110–34.

Rubin, D. H., Leventhal, J. M., Sadock, R. T., Letovsky, E., Schottland, P., Clemente, I., and McCathy, P. 1986. Educational intervention by computer in childhood asthma: a randomized clinical trial testing the use of a new teaching intervention in childhood asthma. *Pediatrics* 77:1–10.

Schneider, S. J., Walter, R., and O'Donnell, R. 1990. Computerized communication as a medium for behavioral smoking cessation treatment: controlled evaluation. *Computers in Human Behavior* 6:141–51.

Selmi, P. M., Klein, M. H., Greist, J. H., Sorrell, S. P., and Erdman, H. P. 1990. Computer-administered cognitive-behavioral therapy for depression. *American Journal of Psychiatry* 147:51–56.

Steuer, J. 1992. Defining virtual reality: dimensions determining telepresence. *Journal of Communication* 42:73–93.

Street, R. L., and Rimal, R. N. 1997. Health promotion and interactive technology: a conceptual foundation. In R. Street and T. Manning, eds., *Using Interactive Computing in Health Promotion*. Rahwah, N.J.: Erlbaum.

Thorkildsen, R., Bickel W. B., and Williams, J. G. 1979. A micro-computer video-disc CAI system for the mentally retarded. *Journal of Special Education Technology* 1:45–51.

Wantland, D. J., Portillo, C. J., Holzemer, W. L., Slaughter, R., and McGhee, E. M. 2004. The effectiveness of web-based vs. non-web-based interventions: a meta-analysis of behavioral change outcomes. *Journal of Medical Internet Research* 6:e40.

Weststone, S. L., Sheehan, T. J., Votaw, R. G., Peterson, M. G., and Rothfield, N. 1985. Evaluation of a computer based education lesson for patients with rheumatoid arthritis. *Journal of Rheumatology* 12:907–12.

Wise, P. H., Dowlatshahi, D. C., Farrant, S., Fromson, S., and Meadows, K. A. 1986. Effect of computer-based learning on diabetes knowledge and control. *Diabetes Care* 9:504–8.

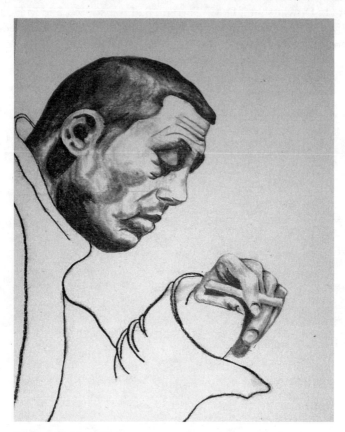

Wayne, by Tina Ennis

4

Office-Based Treatment of Addiction and the Promise of Technology

H. WESTLEY CLARK, M.D., J.D., M.P.H.

As discussed by Dr. Koop in the introductory chapter to this book, it has historically been easy to get addictive drugs and difficult to get treatment. In fact, for many people with opioid addiction, comprehensive treatment including methadone has been geographically out of reach or in settings that were unacceptable. This began to change in 2004 with the national launch of office-based opioid treatment (OBOT)—that is, the potential availability of receiving treatment for opioid addiction in general practice doctors offices nearly anywhere in the nation. As a nation, we still have a long way to go to realize Dr. Koop's vision of treatment being as accessible as addictive drugs, but OBOT is a landmark step in the right direction.

OBOT was made possible by the passage of the Drug Addiction Treatment Act of 2000 (DATA) by the U.S. Congress. DATA not only made OBOT possible but also increased the interest in involving primary care physicians in providing treatment for opioid dependence. Many physicians nevertheless question whether they should be involved in treating opioid-dependent patients. This chapter will address some of the issues, obstacles, and the potential for reform.

Understanding the Magnitude of the Problem

In an effort to estimate the prevalence of opioid abuse in the United States, the National Survey on Drug Use and Health (NSDUH) studied drug use in the general population. On the basis of data collected in 2003, the NSDUH estimated that 3,744,000 individuals had used heroin at least once in their lifetime. A smaller number—314,000—admitted to having used heroin at least once in the past year; and 119,000 admitted to having used heroin in the past month (i.e., are current users). This figure for current users hardly seems to justify mobilizing a cadre of physicians to address the problem, especially because there are more than 1,000 opioid treatment programs in the United States.

Looking at the prevalence of narcotic pain relievers, however, offers another view of the magnitude of opioid use in America. An estimated 31,207,000 Americans admitted to having used opioids for nonmedical purposes at least once in their lifetimes. This number includes 11,671,000 individuals who have used opioids for nonmedical purposes in the past year and 4,693,000 who have done so in the past month (current users).

The number of new initiates to heroin has ranged from 121,000 in 1995 to 164,000 persons in 2002. The number of new initiates to nonmedical use of narcotic pain relievers rose from around 600,000 individuals per year in 1990 to an estimated 2.5 million in 2002.

Data on use alone, however, do not give an adequate picture of the misuse of either heroin or prescription opioid analgesics. The NSDUH estimates that 189,000 individuals meet the criteria for heroin abuse or dependence. Another 1,424,000 individuals meet the criteria for prescription opioid abuse or dependence. Overall about 1.6 million people meet the criteria for abuse or dependence, with the clear majority abusing or being dependent on prescription drugs.

NSDUH data also give some sense of the window of opportunity for intervention for those who abuse prescription drugs. Of those using heroin in the past year, 57.4 percent were classified with abuse or dependence, whereas only 12.2 percent of those using prescription pain relievers met these classifications. Thus, early intervention is critically important for both heroin users and those who abuse prescription pain relievers, but for different reasons. Heroin users often quickly become dependent and thus treatment is rapidly needed. Those who misuse prescription pain relievers appear to generally develop their addictions more gradually, however, delays in intervention mean that there will be more people with problems associated with the misuse of these medications. Intervention would offer both the patient and society a chance of reducing the negative consequences of either heroin use or misuse of prescription pain relievers.

The Capacity of Current Treatment Programs

In light of the magnitude of opioid use across the spectrum from misuse to dependence, the capacity of the substance abuse treatment system to provide access to care for those who need it is important. The Treatment Episode Data Set (TEDS) compiled by the Substance Abuse and Mental Health Services Administration reveals that 331,272 patients were admitted for opioid problems in 2002. This included 285,667 admissions for heroin-related issues and 45,605 admissions for other opioids. Of those treated for opioid-related problems, only 106,944 admissions involved the planned use of methadone, which confirms the observation of many in the field that most people who warrant opioid replacement therapy are not receiving such therapy. This is not to imply that all opioid-dependent persons should receive such therapy or would accept such therapy if it were more readily available; however, the large numbers of potentially eligible people who are not receiving such treatment reinforces other observations that barriers to treatment represent a significant public health challenge.

TEDS does not represent unique individuals; it represents admissions, so it may contain multiple admissions for the same individual. Furthermore, TEDS data do not include admissions to all substance abuse treatment programs, but only those that are licensed or certified by state authorities. Nevertheless, if the TEDS data did represent individuals, then only 20 percent of those who need treatment for opioid-related problems were receiving care through state-recognized substance abuse treatment programs in 2002. Of additional interest is that only 35.2 percent of those admissions for the treatment of heroin and 19.2 percent of those admissions for the treatment of other opiates include methadone as a part of the treatment plan.

In thinking about the treatment system, the first question that must be answered is whether we need medication-assisted therapy for opioid abuse and dependence. The answer is yes. It has been established that psychosocial interventions alone do not work well for the majority of opioid-dependent individuals. In fact, among people receiving methadone, stronger benefits are generally achieved with higher dosages and premature decrease or termination of dosing precipitates relapse (Ball and Ross, 1991). Medication-assisted therapies are an essential element of any strategy to treat opioid abuse and dependence.

As of 2002, there were only 1,080 active medication-assisted opioid treatment programs in the U.S., with an estimated census of 228,000 clients. Six states—Idaho, Montana, Wyoming, North Dakota, South Dakota, and Mississippi—do not have even a single active medication-assisted therapy program. Fifteen other states have fewer than 10 opioid treatment programs within their borders, forcing some clients to travel great distances to receive care.

Office-Based Treatment by Primary Care Providers

Because there is a clear need for medication-assisted treatment for opioid abuse and dependence and a clear shortage of providers to meet that need, any strategy that enhances access to care is desirable. The foremost paradigm available is to involve the practicing physician in her or his office in delivering services to this population in need. The paradigm of an office-based practice includes, of course, physicians who are working in community health clinics.

Before the passage of DATA, methadone and levo-alpha acetyl methadol were the only two drugs readily available for the treatment of opioid abuse and dependence and then only to patients willing to go to tightly regulated clinics or to the rare physician who surmounted the legal, social and economic hurdles to qualify his or her office as a clinic. Hurdles are as diverse as special community approval and zoning permits, costly drug storage facilities, and staffing to meet diverse patient needs—regardless of whether the patient population of a given clinic had all of those needs. Thus, it was not surprising that the overwhelming majority of physicians simply eschewed addressing the problem of opioid abuse and dependence, preferring not to be encumbered by regulatory barriers.

DATA changed that by permitting qualified physicians to use any schedule III, IV, or V medication approved by the Food and Drug Administration (FDA) for the purpose of treating opioid abuse or dependence. In October 2002, the FDA approved buprenorphine for this purpose, thus opening the door for the practicing physician to address opioid abuse or dependence in his or her office. DATA, however, also required physicians who used an office-based model to have the capacity to refer patients for any needed counseling to augment the medication-assisted intervention.

As of October 2004, 3,624 physicians were trained and certified to use buprenorphine for the treatment of opioid abuse and dependence. These physicians are distributed throughout the U.S., with every state having at least one physician with the authority to prescribe buprenorphine on an outpatient basis. Preliminary data indicate, however, that only one-half of physicians certified to use buprenorphine for the treatment of opioid addiction choose to do so.

Thus, incentives are needed to increase the number of physicians certified to treat opioid-abusing or -dependent patients. Before creating appropriate incentives, we need to understand why certified physicians are not providing care to these individuals.

Taking Advantage of Information Technology in the Treatment of Opioid Dependence

One assumption is that a lack of familiarity with the patient population and with the treatment strategies needed for a positive outcome discourages many physicians. Electronic medicine or telemedicine may offer the addiction field an opportunity to assist the primary care physician or general psychiatrist in extending clinical care to addicted patients. Computer-based consultation with experts in the addiction field through Internet listservs, instant messaging, chat rooms, or e-mail permits physicians to find information about clinical strategies quickly. Although abundant literature is available on the use of telepsychiatry in clinics, hospitals, group homes, homeless shelters, schools, and forensic facilities, the necessary equipment required for using it is costly. It is unlikely that physicians ambivalent about treating addiction would be willing to invest in specific teleconferencing technology packages; however, in light of declining costs of both computers and broadband access, a major limitation associated with telemedicine could be eliminated. Using Internet technology, organized groups of providers or experts could mentor and/or consult with physicians less experienced in treating addiction.

Assuring appropriate access to counseling is another challenge that information technology can help address. One issue that confronts some physicians in general practice (primary care or general psychiatry), particularly those who practice in rural areas, is the inability to make appropriate referrals for addiction counseling. Since the workforce shortages adversely affect access to traditional substance abuse services, it may be necessary for the physician community to incorporate new technologies in their treatment planning. Electronic medicine—including electronic assessment and therapy and computer-assisted behavioral health care—offers the office-based practitioner an opportunity to help opioid-abusing or -dependent patients access care that would otherwise be unavailable. The use of technology can augment the reach of individual practitioners or of health clinics unfamiliar with addiction or co-occurring substance use and mental health disorders. Thus, in this paradigm, technology could enhance physicians' skills and also benefit patients.

Telemedicine-based clinical strategies depend on the technology being accessible to both the professional seeking skill enhancement and the patient seeking care. Although computers are increasingly essential for physicians, they may remain out of financial reach for many patients. For patients without home-based information systems, access points to electronic information could be established in several locations such as libraries, community health centers, and community centers. Patients with substance abuse or addiction problems might find a more responsive health care practitioner or a more welcoming environment online than in face-to-face meetings at a health clinic. Although challenges associated with electronic assessment and therapy such as patient acceptance, confidentiality, quality of service, certification, and licensure issues still need to be addressed and resolved, electronic medicine is a valuable method to provide health care information and access to treatment.

Opoid abuse and dependence are clearly undertreated in the U.S. Novel approaches are needed. Office-based treatment of addiction is one promising possibility, and information technology can help make that promise a common reality.

REFERENCES

Ball, J. C., and Ross, A. 1991. *The Effectiveness of Methadone Maintenance Treatment.* New York: Springer-Verlag.

5

High-Impact Paradigms for the Treatment of Addiction

JAMES O. PROCHASKA, PH.D.

Addiction treatments in the twenty-first century need to be evaluated by impact rather than efficacy. Currently, impact = (efficacy × reach). In the twentieth century, a treatment with 30 percent efficacy (e.g., abstinence) was judged to be 50 percent better than a treatment with 20 percent efficacy, but if the first treatment reaches only 5 percent of an addicted population, it produces only a 1.5 percent impact (30 percent × 5 percent) on prevalence of addiction in that population. In comparison, a treatment that has only 20 percent efficacy but reaches 75 percent of a population has 15 percent impact. The treatment with lower efficacy has 10 times more impact. To dramatically increase the impact of addiction treatments, traditional paradigms of practice and research must be complemented by innovative paradigms (Prochaska, 2004).

Innovative Paradigms for Addiction Treatment

Individual Patient Paradigm Complemented by Population Paradigm. Traditional treatments focus primarily on individual patients who seek services and ignore the multitude who do not. When managed care organizations offer action-oriented smoking cessation clinics for free, removing cost as a barrier, only about 1 percent of eligible smokers participate. No wonder comprehensive tobacco control programs have emphasized social policies (like taxes) and environmental controls (like bans in public places). Policies are population based, whereas treatments have not been (Prochaska and Velicer, 2004).

Passive-Reactive Paradigm Complemented by Outreach Paradigm. Clinicians have been socialized to wait passively for patients to seek services and then they react. Passive-reactive practices are designed to treat acute conditions in patients with acute pain, distress, or illness. With some deadly addictions like smoking, however, most patients are not yet experiencing acute pain, distress, or illness. Clinicians need to think of these behaviors as silent killers—like hypertension—and they need to assess and treat such addictions proactively the way they do hypertension. Proactive outreach to adolescent and adult smokers from primary care practices, to students on campus who abuse alcohol, and to populations with problems ranging from obesity, stress, and inactivity to bullying have consistently produced recruitment rates of 65 to 85 percent.

Action Paradigm Complemented by Stage Paradigm. When a high percentage of populations participate in treatment, the large majority will not be prepared to take immediate action. Among smokers in the United States, about 20 percent are prepared to quit in the next month; among alcohol abusers on campus, that figure is about 10 percent. Among the 300 million smokers in China, about 5 percent are prepared to quit and more than 70 percent are in the precontemplation stage and are not intending to take action in the next six months. Relying on action-oriented interventions will fail to provide appropriate treatment for the majority of such populations.

Efficacy Paradigm Complemented by Effectiveness Paradigm. In developing the most recent clinical practice guidelines for treatment of tobacco dependence (Fiore et al., 2000), Fiore and colleagues had access to more than 6,000 studies on tobacco. From the best of the reported randomized clinical efficacy trials, the guidelines identified an impressive range of evidence-based treatments for smokers who are prepared to quit in the next month, but they identified no evidence-based treatments for the 80 percent of smokers who are not motivated to quit. Efficacy trials are highly selective, recruiting homogeneous participant populations, such as smokers who are motivated to quit or who are free from mental illness problems. Consequently, the guidelines incorporate no evidence-based treatments for smokers with mental illness, even though 47 percent of all cigarettes are purchased by such smokers.

In contrast, effectiveness trials are population based and are typically designed to reach as broad and heterogeneous a group as possible. Efficacy trials that exclude the vast majority of addicted populations cannot continue to be the primary evidence base if addiction treatments are to have dramatically increased impacts.

Clinic Paradigm Complemented by Self-Management Paradigm. For most primary care, patients administer treatment at home themselves. This is a major reason why primary care relies so heavily on pharmaceuticals. Most patients do not want clinic-based treatments. For example, marketing research with obese and overweight populations in the U.S. has found that only about 5 percent want clinic- or group-based treatments; 50 percent want home-based care. With some of the highest risk, most costly of chronic conditions, such as diabetes, disease management companies proactively reach out to populations at home by telephone to help them change behaviors and improve self-management.

Clinician Paradigm Complemented by Computer Paradigm. Almost all of our proactive population and stage-based effectiveness trials have relied heavily on individualized communications generated by computers driven by expert systems. Participants complete clinical assessments by telephone, mail, or Internet and then receive expert guidance that provides feedback on what processes and principles of behavior change they are applying appropriately and what mistakes they are making. Such systems have produced significant impacts at 12- to 24-month follow-up, including rates of abstinence of about 25 percent among diverse populations, such as adolescent, adult, and depressed smokers (Prochaska et al., 2001a, 2001b; Hollis et al., 2005). To date, adding proactive telephone counselors to computer-generated communications have failed to increase efficacy. Interactive technologies are likely to be to behavior medicine what pharmaceuticals are to biological medicine, namely, a cost-effective approach to deliver optimal care to enhance health in populations at home with few or no side effects.

Single Behavior Paradigm Complemented by Multiple Behaviors Paradigm. The highest-risk and highest-cost populations, like those with addictions, have multiple behavior problems, but most of our clinical knowledge is based on single behavior studies. The established clinical wisdom is to treat only one behavior at a time lest clients (and clinicians?) be overwhelmed by too many demands. Substance abuse treatment, for example, would typically not touch smoking because patients were assumed to need something to help them cope with stress and distress, but a recent meta-analysis found that patients did better with their primary substance abuse when they were also treated for smoking (Prochaska et al., 2004a).

In a growing series of disease-prevention and disease-management trials involving multiple behavior changes, participants were as successful quitting smoking when they were treated for three or four behaviors simultaneously as were those who were treated just for smoking (22 percent to 26 percent abstinent at 12 to 24 months). They were even more successful with the other treated behaviors, such as diet and self-monitoring of blood glucose for self-management of diabetes (Jones et al., 2003; Prochaska et al., 2004b). Multiple behavior changes, however, have greater impact on health and health care costs. A new equation would be: impact = (efficacy × reach × number of behaviors changed).

Toward an Inclusive Care Model for Addictions

Integrating just one or two innovative paradigms will not produce nearly as much impact as integrating the entire cluster. One of the most intensive proactive protocols in the literature had a sequence of physicians, nurses, health educator, and telephone counselors reach out to all smokers to get them to sign up for action-oriented clinics. They were able to get 35 percent of smokers in the precontemplation stage to sign up, but only 3 percent actually showed up for treatment (Lichtenstein and Hollis, 1992). With home-based, action-oriented telephone support lines ("quit lines"), states typically budget for one-quarter of 1 percent of smokers calling these passive-reactive quit lines, which are designed for highly motivated smokers who are prepared to quit in the next week.

All of these innovative paradigms are designed to be as inclusive as possible. Heterogeneous effectiveness trials, for example, are much more inclusive than selective efficacy trials that exclude unmotivated patients or patients with co-morbidities. Multiple behavior paradigms, by definition, include more target behaviors than do single behavior paradigms, and proactive practices reach much higher percentages of populations than do traditional passive reactive approaches.

This is not to say that the traditional paradigms do not play an important role in the treatment of addictions and other health behaviors. Such science and services are critical for individual patients who are motivated or prepared to participate in such programs. They must be complemented by innovative paradigms to reach the significant percentages of populations who have not been studied or served in the past. A mission for the future is to combine more inclusive science with more inclusive services to produce more inclusive care that can have much greater effects on chronic conditions like the addictions.

REFERENCES

Fiore, M. C., Bailey, W. C., Cohen, S. J., Dorfman, S. F., Goldstein, M. G., Gritz, E. R., Heyman, R. B., Jaén, C. R., Kottke, T. E., Lando, H. A., Mecklenburg, R. E., Mullen, P. D., Nett, L. M., Robinson, L., Stitzer, M. L., Tommasello, A. C., Villejo, L., and Wewers, M. E. 2000. *Treating Tobacco Use and Dependence: Clinical Practice Guideline*. Rockville, Md.: U.S. Department of Health and Human Services, Public Health Service.

Hollis, J. F., Polen, M. R., Whitlock, E. P., Lichtenstein, E., Mullooly, J. P., Velicer, W. F., and Redding, C. A. 2005. Teen REACH: outcomes from a randomized controlled trial of tobacco reduction program for teens seen in primary medical care. *Pediatrics* 114:981–9.

Jones, H., Edwards, L., Vallis, T. M., Ruggiero, L., Rossi, S. R, Rossi, J. S., Greene, G., Prochaska, J. O., and Zinman, B. 2003. Changes in diabetes self-care behaviors make a difference in glycemic control: the Diabetes Stages of Change (DiSC) study. *Diabetes Care* 26:1468–74.

Prochaska, J. O. 2004. Population treatment for addictions. *Current Directions in Psychological Science* 13:242–46.

Prochaska, J .O., and Velicer, W. F. 2004. Integrating population smoking cessation policies and programs. Public Health Reports. *Journal of the U.S. Public Health Service* 119 (special issue, May–June):244–52.

Prochaska, J. O., Velicer, W. F., Fava, J. L., Rossi, J. S., and Tsoh, J. Y. 2001a. Evaluating a population-based recruitment approach and stage-based expert system intervention for smoking cessation. *Addictive Behaviors* 26:583–602.

Prochaksa, J. O., Velicer, W. F., Fava, J. L., Ruggiero, L., Laforge, R. G., Rossi, J. S., Johnson, S. S., and Lee, P. A. 2001b. Counselor and stimulus control enhancements for a stage-matched expert system for smokers in a managed care setting. *Preventive Medicine* 32:23–32.

Prochaska, J. O., Delucchi, K., and Hall, S. M. 2004a. A meta-analysis of smoking cessation interventions with individuals in substance abuse treatment or recovery. *Journal of Consulting and Clinical Psychology* 72:1144–56.

Prochaska, J. O., Velicer, W. F., Rossi, J. S., Redding, C. A., Greene, G. W., Rossi, S. R., Sun, X., Fava, J. L., Laforge, R. G., and Plummer, B. 2004b. Multiple risk expert systems interventions: impact of simultaneous stage-matched expert systems for multiple behaviors in a population of parents. *Health Psychology* 2:503–16.

6

New Approaches to the Treatment of Stimulant and Other Substance Abuse
A Behavioral Perspective

MAXINE L. STITZER, PH.D.

Stimulant abuse continues to be a major problem in the United States and worldwide, as evidenced by population survey data and treatment admissions (Community Epidemiology Work Group, 2004). The drugs in this class—including cocaine, crack cocaine, and methamphetamine—continue to be widely available in the United States, with the result that an estimated 2.3 million people are current users of cocaine, while about 1.3 million are users of methamphetamine (National Survey on Drug Use and Health, 2003). Stimulant abusers are found in psychosocial counseling programs, where they may be undergoing treatment of primary stimulant abuse or mixed abuse of stimulants plus alcohol and/or marijuana. A substantial number of stimulant abusers are also found in methadone maintenance programs, where their use of stimulants may continue during treatment.

Although pharmacotherapy is included in some programs, there has not yet been a pharmacotherapeutic approach for stimulant abuse widely proven or used as, for example, methadone and buprenorphine approaches for opioid dependence. This has fostered active development and evaluation of behavioral approaches. Focusing on basic principles of behavior suggests several new directions for the ideal content and structure of treatment interventions for stimulant abusers. This behavioral focus has potential to further improve treatment of substance abuse and dependence to drugs other than stimulants.

Counteracting Potent and Immediate Drug Reinforcers

A basic premise of drug abuse treatment is that the treatment intervention must compete for the attention (and behavior) of the abuser with the powerful and immediate reinforcing effects of their favorite drug(s). Drugs exert a compelling force, luring the abuser back to the remembered pleasures and comforts of use even during periods of stable abstinence. Because of the lure of potent drug reinforcers, it is realistic to assume that the motivation of drug abusers to stop their use of stimulants may be low overall and that motivation may fluctuate over time as the negative consequences of drug use become more or less salient. The tools available to treatment providers in this competition with drug reinforcers are few; treatment of stimulant abuse poses a unique challenge because there are no medications available to help with the task. Thus, treatment of stimulant abuse traditionally relies heavily on the natural features of the abuser's environment that have prompted him or her to enter treatment, on the persuasive power of the client-counselor interaction, and on teaching new skills to help clients effectively avoid drug use and build a satisfying, drug-free lifestyle. The following sections discuss some specific areas where behavioral principles might be usefully employed to further improve treatment for stimulant abuse.

Reducing Response Cost for Treatment Entry

Response cost for treatment entry—that is, the difficulties and barriers encountered by individuals who want to enter treatment programs—is the first place to look for new approaches that might improve overall success of the treatment system in dealing with stimulant abusers. Reducing the response cost for entering treatment by making it easier for individuals to enter and stay in treatment programs might be considered as a way to increase rates of treatment entry. One example of a way to make treatment more accessible would be to use mobile vans or community-based sites for treatment delivery rather than requiring that those in treatment make their way repeatedly to fixed-site clinics. An innovative mobile van methadone project in Baltimore exemplifies this approach (Greenfield et al., 1996; Kuo et al., 2003). Another approach that could reduce response cost would be to streamline the traditional intake process, which typically involves several demanding hours of intrusive, often repetitive, questioning. Reducing the intake response cost might plausibly be expected to increase the number of people who apply to treatment. Thus, taking steps to reduce response cost could increase the likelihood that stimulant abusers will enter treatment in the first place. Reducing response cost might also reduce the number of individuals who complete intake but fail to return for subsequently scheduled clinic visits, a problem that is especially apparent in psychosocial counseling programs.

Using Alternative Reinforcement to Counter Treatment Dropout

Motivating clients to stay in treatment is a second key consideration in drug abuse treatment. This is not so much an issue in methadone treatment, because the methadone medication itself appears sufficiently reinforcing to sustain reasonably good retention. In psychosocial counseling programs, however, 20 percent or fewer patients may be retained through a six-month treatment program (McKay, 2001). Providing an attractive, engaging treatment program with ample social reinforcement could certainly help to improve retention. Using explicit, tangible incentives in the form of vouchers or prizes contingent on clinic attendance, however, may also be a useful strategy. One recently completed multisite clinical trial that offered prize incentives for drug-free urine samples to stimulant (cocaine or methamphetamine) abusers enrolled in psychosocial counseling programs found a significant improvement in retention (Petry et al., 2005). Among those who could earn prizes, there was a 50 percent retention rate over 12 weeks compared with 35 percent retention among participants enrolled in the usual care control arm. These results suggest that adoption of incentive procedures should be seriously considered as a routine part of care in psychosocial counseling programs as a means to improve treatment retention. It is possible that incentives directly targeting attendance rather than drug abstinence might be effective in achieving this goal.

Using Alternative Reinforcement
to Counter Drug Use during Treatment

A third key objective of drug abuse treatment is to initiate and support continuing abstinence from drugs. The principle of alternative reinforcement has been effectively brought to bear in drug abuse treatment to counter the persistent lure of potent drug reinforcers that underlies cycles of drug use and relapse. Voucher and prize-based reinforcement systems targeting drug abstinence have repeatedly been shown in controlled research to be an efficacious intervention for promoting sustained abstinence with stimulant abusers enrolled in psychosocial counseling programs (Higgins et al., 1994, 2000). Emerging evidence indicates that, among stimulant abusers who are also methadone patients, both aversive control, in the form of threats to discontinue the treatment episode (Brooner et al., 1998; McCarthy and Borders, 1985), and positive reinforcement, in the form of abstinence incentive programs offering methadone take-home privileges, monetary vouchers (Silverman et al., 1996, 1998, 2004), and prizes (Petry and Martin, 2002), have been shown to be efficacious for reducing during-treatment stimulant (cocaine) use. This finding has recently been replicated in a large sample, multisite clinical trial from the National Drug Abuse Treatment Clinical Trials Network (Peirce et al., 2006) in which the incentive doubled the likelihood that a stimulant-negative urine sample would be submitted. Taken together, these studies support the further adoption of incentive-based treatment approaches into community methadone treatment programs among other standard care options intended to strengthen treatment effectiveness.

Developing Stepped Care Models
to Accommodate Individual Differences

A final challenge to the design and delivery of drug abuse treatment is the need to accommodate and address individual differences in response to treatment interventions. There are large individual differences in the ability of drug abusers to accept the demands of even the best treatments, including abstinence reinforcement interventions. For example, only about 50–60 percent of individuals offered vouchers or prizes for drug-free urine samples typically respond well and initiate long periods of abstinence, even when the potential value of the rewards is substantial (Silverman et al., 1996, 2004). Stepped-care models could offer options for individuals who are resistant to treatment. In some cases, it may be necessary to alter only the type or magnitude of alternative reinforcers offered for therapeutic behavior change. In other cases, it may be necessary for the treatment program to take steps to alter adverse settings (e.g., housing situations) that contribute to maintenance of drug use (e.g., Jason et al., 2007). Ultimately, a stepped-care model could include structured residential environments (sometimes referred to as "synthetic environments") in which drug abusers who have difficulty abstaining in their usual environment are removed from the stimulus control of people and places that have supported their drug use. In such an environment, individuals could learn new skills and be exposed to new, alternative reinforcers that may improve their chances of resuming a productive and drug-free lifestyle on completion of intensive treatment.

For example, incarceration routinely removes drug abusers from the cues formerly associated with drug use, and thus prisons could be a good setting in which to implement effective rehabilitation programs for drug abusers. Furthermore, there is currently a resurgence of interest in prison-based treatment. In light of the large numbers of incarcerated individuals with drug abuse problems, this would seem like an efficient use of resources, provided that prison-based programs are coordinated with appropriate support in the community following release.

Developing Chronic Disease Management Models of Treatment

A fundamental characteristic of drug abuse is that it is a chronic relapsing disorder, an observation that appears to call for a change in the way we conceptualize treatment. Treatment is currently conceptualized within an "inoculation" model, in which drug abusers come to a program, learn something new, and leave as changed people inspired and equipped for recovery. In view of the recognition that drug abuse is a chronic relapsing disorder, however, there is a need to recognize the potential utility of a treatment model that incorporates continuing care over prolonged periods of time. Routine, periodic checkups following an acute care episode could serve to identify those individuals who are beginning to slip back into drug use, and interventions could be put in place to re-engage these individuals in additional treatment to forestall full relapse and return them to an abstinent state. The idea of continuing care with repeat treatment episodes is one that is just beginning to be explored (e.g., McKay, 2001; Godley et al., 2002; Dennis et al., 2003), and considerable effort would be needed to develop the right interventions to entice drug abusers back repeatedly into treatment. Nevertheless, this could be a potentially important future direction.

Identifying Characteristics of Ideal Treatment Programs

Further research is needed to identify characteristics of ideal drug abuse treatment programs. Drug abuse treatment is a complex and multifaceted enterprise. It incorporates many structural (e.g., clinic size and location, expected duration and frequency of treatment), contextual (treatment modality and philosophy), and interpersonal (leadership and counselor) influences, in addition to the specific types of interventions that may be implemented with greater or lesser competence by therapists. Thus, it is daunting to envision isolating and studying treatment factors in controlled research. This is nevertheless exactly what needs to happen to better shape and inform the treatment delivery system. One approach might be to develop a standardized treatment protocol (i.e., with fixed, clearly defined parameters) to be used as a comparison condition in research. It would be of interest to compare outcomes across several clinics that used the same standardized protocol to assess variability due to patient characteristics and other factors that are not controlled within the standardized protocol. It would also be of interest to compare outcomes for the standardized protocol with those of other usual care programs to see how well the standardized protocol performs. Baseline performance would ideally be such that either improvements or decrements could be detected. Finally, elements of treatment structure and/or content could be systematically varied to provide persuasive evidence for the value of different treatment parameters or innovations.

Overall, the development and delivery of drug abuse treatment services in the U.S. and worldwide made enormous strides in the closing decades of the twentieth century. The incorporation of behavioral principles and knowledge from treatment research more generally into services delivery and community practice, however, remains within the province of relatively few treatment programs. Of course, continuing research is vital to address the challenges posed by the need to reliably counter potent drug reinforcers to support long-term abstinence and meet the needs of people who are refractory to even the best of currently available treatments. Continuing to explore behavioral, social, and physiological mediators of drug addiction, including its chronic relapsing nature and individual differences in response to treatment interventions, will be essential for continuing to develop new, more effective treatment. As the foregoing discussion indicates, principles of behavior can provide a highly useful theoretical framework for conceptualizing both drug abuse and development of therapies for stimulant abusers. The field will no doubt do well to continue to use this perspective to inform future research and development. These advances make the possibility of managing drug addiction, at least as well as other major disorders such as hypertension, depression, and diabetes (all of which include behavioral and pharmacological interventions), a realistic goal for the twenty-first century.

REFERENCES

Community Epidemiology Work Group. 2004. *Epidemiologic Trends in Drug Abuse*. Vol. 1: *Proceedings of the Community Epidemiology Work Group*. Washington, D.C.: U.S. Department of Health and Human Services.

Brooner, R. K., Kidorf, M., King, V. L., and Stoller, K. 1998. Preliminary evidence of good treatment response in antisocial drug abusers. *Drug and Alcohol Dependence* 49:249–60.

Dennis, M. L., Scott, C. K., and Funk, R. 2003. Main findings from an experimental evaluation of recovery management checkups and early re-intervention (RMC/ERI) with chronic substance users. *Evaluation and Program Planning* 26:339–52.

Godley, M. D., Godley, S. H., Dennis, M. L., Funk, R., and Passetti, L. 2002. Preliminary outcomes from the assertive continuing care experiment for adolescents discharged from residential treatment. *Journal of Substance Abuse Treatment* 23:21–32.

Greenfield, L., Brady, J. V., Besteman, K. J., and De Smet, A. 1996. Patient retention in mobile and fixed-site methadone maintenance treatment. *Drug and Alcohol Dependence* 42:125–31.

Higgins, S. T., Budney, A. J., Bickel, W. K., Foerg, F. E., Donham, R., and

Badger, G. J. 1994. Incentives improve outcome in outpatient behavioral treatment of cocaine dependence. *Archives of General Psychiatry* 51:568–76.

Higgins, S. T., Wong, C. J., Badger, G. J., Ogden, D. E., and Dantona, R. A. 2000. Contingent reinforcement increases cocaine abstinence during outpatient treatment and 1 year of follow-up. *Journal of Consulting and Clinical Psychology* 68:64–72.

Jason, L. A., Olson, B. D., Ferrari, J. R., Majer, J. M., Alvarez, J., and Stout, J. 2007. An examination of main and interactive effects of substance abuse recovery housing on multiple indicators of adjustment. *Addiction* 102:1114–1121.

Kuo, I., Brady, J., Butler, C., Schwartz, R., Brooner, R., Vlahov, D., and Strathdee, S. A. 2003. Feasibility of referring drug users from a needle exchange program into an addiction treatment program: experience with a mobile treatment van and LAAM maintenance. *Journal of Substance Abuse Treatment* 24:67–74.

McCarthy, J. J., and Borders, O. T. 1985. Limit setting on drug abuse in methadone maintenance patients. *American Journal of Psychiatry* 142:1419–23.

McKay, J. R. 2001. Effectiveness of continuing care interventions for substance abusers: implications for the study of long-term effects. *Evaluation Review* 25:211–32.

National Survey on Drug Use and Health, 2003. Substance Abuse and Mental Health Services Administration (SAMHSA). U.S. Department of Health and Human Services. www.samhsa.gov.

Peirce, J. M., Petry, N. M., Stitzer, M. L., Blaine, J., Kellogg, S., Satterfield, F., Schwartz, M., Krasnansky, J., Pencer, E., Silva-Vasquez, L., Kirby, K. C., Royer-Malvestuto, C., Roll, J. M., Cohen, A., Copersino, M. L., Kolodner, K., and Li, R. 2006. Effects of lower-cost incentives on stimulant abstinence in methadone maintenance treatment: a National Drug Abuse Treatment Clinical Trials Network study. *Archives of General Psychiatry* 63:201–8.

Petry, N. M., and Martin, B. 2002. Low-cost contingency management for treating cocaine- and opioid-abusing methadone patients. *Journal of Consulting and Clinical Psychology* 70:398–405.

Petry, N. M., Peirce, J. M., Stitzer, M. L., Blaine, J., Roll, J. M., Cohen, A., Obert, J., Killeen, T., Saladin, M. E., Cowell, M., Kirby, K. C., Sterling, R., Royer-Malvestuto, C., Hamilton, J., Booth, R. E., Macdonald, M., Liebert, M., Rader, L., Burns, R., DiMaria, J., Copersino, M., Stabile, P. Q., Kolodner, K., and Li, R. 2005. Effect of prize-based incentives on outcomes in stimulant abusers in outpatient psychosocial treatment programs: a national drug abuse treatment clinical trials network study. *Archives of General Psychiatry* 23:1148–56.

Silverman, K., Robles, E., Mudric, T., Bigelow, G. E., and Stitzer, M. L. 2004. A randomized trial of long-term reinforcement of cocaine abstinence in methadone-maintained patients who inject drugs. *Journal of Consulting and Clinical Psychology* 72:839–54.

Silverman, K., Wong, C. J., Umbricht-Schneiter, A., Montoya, I. D., Schuster, C. R., and Preston, K. L. 1998. Broad beneficial effects of cocaine abstinence reinforcement among methadone patients. *Journal of Consulting and Clinical Psychology* 66:811–24.

Silverman, K., Higgins, S. T., Brooner, R. K., Montoya, I. D., Cone, E. J., Schuster, C. R., and Preston, K. L. 1996. Sustained cocaine abstinence in methadone maintenance patients through voucher-based reinforcement therapy. *Archives of General Psychiatry* 53:409–15.

7

Using Diminished Autonomy over Tobacco Use to Identify Smokers in Need of Assistance with Cessation

JOSEPH R. DIFRANZA, M.D.

Before graduating from medical school in 1981, I was taught that one had to smoke for years to be hooked. The prevailing assumption was that years of practice and repetition engendered habitual smoking; with tolerance developing insidiously. On the assumption that dependence was a consequence of tolerance, it began only after prolonged daily smoking of at least five cigarettes per day. Limiting consumption to fewer than five cigarettes per day or nondaily smoking was assumed by many to confer a safe refuge from dependence. Withdrawal would be absent in those who did not smoke every day. A seasoned smoking-cessation counselor advised that adolescents did not need cessation help because they were not hooked. Although medicine was not primitive in 1981—it had been more than a decade since the first heart transplant—everything I learned in medical school about the onset of tobacco dependence was wrong.

To begin with, not a single study supports the belief that withdrawal symptoms are entirely absent among those who do not smoke daily. To the contrary, at least 12 studies report withdrawal symptoms prior to the initiation of daily smoking. Nor are smokers who experience withdrawal symptoms bound to smoking at least five cigarettes each day: a single cigarette can keep withdrawal symptoms at bay for two to three days in nondaily smokers (DiFranza et al., 2000, 2002a). Although individuals who have nurtured a substantial tolerance to nicotine may have to maintain minimum nicotine levels to avoid withdrawal, this is certainly not true of nondaily smokers.

Withdrawal is not the only symptom of dependence that appears quickly. Some individuals warrant a diagnosis of nicotine dependence prior to the onset of daily smoking, either by the criteria of the World Health Organization or the American Psychiatric Association in their diagnostic manuals. For example, symptoms of dependence, such as craving and withdrawal, were observed at an average smoking rate of only two cigarettes per week (DiFranza et al., 2000, 2002b). This implies that tolerance, in terms of moderate to heavy smoking, is not the cause of dependence. Indeed, in a prospective study, the escalation of consumption beyond two cigarettes per day occurred almost exclusively in smokers who already had dependence symptoms (Wellman et al., 2004). Tolerance appears to be a consequence of tobacco dependence rather than its cause.

Perhaps because of the negative connotations of the label "drug addict," conventional criteria for a diagnosis of nicotine dependence emphasize the presence of the often long-term, self-destructive sequelae of substance use. This approach has obvious limitations for assessing when and how dependence starts, or for identifying which smokers might require some assistance with cessation.

An alternative approach is to assess autonomy—that is, the freedom to not smoke. Autonomy is diminished when the physical or psychological sequelae of tobacco use present an obstacle to cessation (Wellman et al., 2005). Diminished autonomy does not make quitting impossible, but it does make it more difficult or unpleasant. The Hooked on Nicotine Checklist (HONC) was constructed from ten survey items that have face validity as indicators of diminished autonomy (Table 7.1). The HONC has demonstrated a good to excellent level of internal reliability in both adolescents and adults, and autonomy as measured by the HONC has proved to be a better predictor of continued use than either the more widely used Fagerstrom Test for Nicotine Dependence or the American Psychiatric Association's diagnostic criteria (DiFranza et al., 2000, 2002b).

The HONC was developed as a tool for studying the onset of dependence. Prospective studies indicate that symptoms of diminished autonomy can develop in novice smokers within days of the onset of intermittent smoking (DiFranza et al., 2002b). Contradicting conven-

Table 7.1. The Hooked on Nicotine Checklist

1. Have you ever tried to quit smoking, but couldn't?
2. Do you smoke now because it is hard to quit?
3. Have you ever felt you were addicted to tobacco?
4. Do you ever have strong cravings to smoke?
5. Have you ever felt you really needed a cigarette?
6. Is it hard to keep from smoking in places where you are not supposed to, such as school?

When you tried to stop smoking (or when you haven't used tobacco for a while):

7. Did you find it hard to concentrate because you couldn't smoke?
8. Did you feel more irritable because you couldn't smoke?
9. Did you feel a strong need or urge to smoke?
10. Did you feel nervous, restless, or anxious because you couldn't smoke?

Source: DiFranza et al. (2002b).

tional wisdom, symptoms can be present before novice smokers learn to look natural holding a cigarette, or develop habits. Each of the ten symptoms of diminished autonomy that form the items of the HONC (Table 7.1) has been reported before the onset of daily smoking. Failed attempts at cessation are surprisingly common among youths who have not progressed to daily smoking. Youths who had not yet smoked 20 cigarettes (one pack) reported failed cessation attempts (Barker, 1994). The number of HONC symptoms correlates well with levels of cigarette consumption in both adolescents and adults; however, when adolescents are compared to adults who smoke the same number of cigarettes, adolescents have significantly more symptoms of diminished autonomy. Because dependence develops before tolerance, adolescents are far more dependent than would be expected based on the number of cigarettes they smoke.

To summarize, mounting evidence indicates that diminished autonomy over tobacco can occur soon after the onset of intermittent use and is usually present by the time individuals are smoking only one cigarette per day. Even early symptoms of diminished autonomy are strong predictors of the future trajectory of smoking. A positive response to at least one question on the HONC was strongly predictive of a failed attempt at cessation, and continued smoking over time

(DiFranza et al., 2002b). Russell estimated that more than 90 percent of youths who smoke three to four cigarettes will become addicted and smoke for many years (Russell, 1990). The rapid development of diminished autonomy at low levels of consumption is consistent with his observation. Those who question whether adolescents have an interest in quitting should be aware of data from six surveys which reveal that between 71 and 83 percent have experienced a failed quit attempt; many make repeated attempts, but typically it takes someone who began smoking in adolescence decades to quit (Pierce and Gilpin, 1996).

Whether these obstacles are surmountable by an individual depends on many factors, such as his or her emotional coping skills, social support, prior cessation experience, and access to professional advice and pharmacological aides. We do not know that it is any easier for a 14-year-old high school freshman who smokes three cigarettes per week to quit than it is for a 40-year-old teacher who smokes a pack per day and has made multiple previous attempts. Although the obstacles that adolescents face are possibly of lesser magnitude than those of adults who have smoked for many years, so too are the resources available to them to overcome those obstacles.

At any level of use, the hazards of tobacco far outweigh any benefits. Because there is no safe level of use, the standard of care is to advise all smokers to quit, and the sooner the better. There is no reason to wait until an official diagnosis of tobacco dependence can be made before offering help. An individual may not meet diagnostic criteria and yet still need help with cessation.

The loss of autonomy is a core feature of dependence to all drugs of abuse. Smokers who attempt cessation are trying to regain their autonomy over tobacco use. A measure of diminished autonomy has certain advantages over other measures of dependence, such as the Fagerstrom Tolerance Questionnaire or the American Psychiatric Association criteria, because it identifies the key reasons why individuals need help with cessation. We should resist the tendency to withhold treatment until the problem meets major diagnostic criteria. Early treatment is more successful. All smokers who report diminished autonomy over tobacco should be offered cessation help regardless of how little they smoke.

REFERENCES

Barker, D. 1994. Reasons for tobacco use and symptoms of nicotine withdrawal among adolescent and young adult tobacco users, United States, 1993. *Morbidity and Mortality Weekly Report* 43:745–50.

DiFranza, J. R., Rigotti, N. A., McNeill, A. D., Ockene, J. K., Savageau, J. A., St Cyr, D., and Coleman, M. 2000. Initial symptoms of nicotine dependence in adolescents. *Tobacco Control* 9:313–19.

DiFranza, J. R., Savageau, J. A., Fletcher, K., Ockene, J. K., Rigotti, N. A., McNeill, A. D., Coleman, M., and Wood, C. 2002a. The development of symptoms of tobacco dependence in youths: 30-month follow-up data from the DANDY study. *Tobacco Control* 11:228–35.

DiFranza, J. R., Savageau, J.A., Fletcher, K., Ockene, J. K., Rigotti, N. A., McNeill, A. D., Coleman, M., and Wood, C. 2002b. Measuring the loss of autonomy over nicotine use in adolescents: The DANDY Development and Assessment of Nicotine Dependence in Youths (DANDY) Study. *Archives of Pediatric and Adolescent Medicine* 156:397–403.

Pierce, J. P., and Gilpin, E. 1996. How long will today's new adolescent smoker be addicted to cigarettes? *American Journal of Public Health* 86:253–56.

Russell, M. A. H. 1990. The nicotine addiction trap: a 40-year sentence for four cigarettes. *British Journal of Addiction* 85:293–300.

Wellman, R. J., DiFranza, J. R., Savageau, J.A., and Dussault, G.F. 2004. Short-term patterns of early smoking acquisition. *Tobacco Control* 13:251–57.

Wellman, R. J., DiFranza, J. R., Savageau, J. A., Godiwala, S., Friedman, K., and Hazelton, J. 2005. Measuring adults' loss of autonomy over nicotine use: The Hooked on Nicotine Checklist. *Nicotine and Tobacco Research* 7:157–61.

8

New Directions for Tobacco Cessation Therapies

EDWARD F. DOMINO, M.D.

Humans have been using tobacco products for at least 4,000 years. One of the lessons from this long history, no matter what the culture or society using tobacco, is that in spite of costs and penalties many chronic users have great difficulty in quitting. A new view is needed if we are to address this problem successfully.

To date, public policy efforts have not effectively supported interventions to help all who need treatment. No legislative body has yet provided enough funds for all of the necessary educational, medical, and psychological support for smokers who wish to quit. Just seven years into the twenty-first century, it requires only a cursory review of the literature to identify the inadequacies of current therapeutic interventions used to achieve long-term tobacco cessation.

The 1990s master settlement agreement against the tobacco industry provided 206 billion dollars to states but has provided little overall treatment support to tobacco users because state governments have used many of the funds for other needs, such as repairing roads, funding life science or high-tech company initiatives, or simply balancing general budgets. If such use of those funds continues, it will insure the existence of a profitable tobacco industry for at least the next two decades.

Feldman and Bayer (2004) reviewed the history of tobacco control policies of eight nations, including members of the European Union. Their research showed clearly that tobacco control by members of the

European Union depends more on trade and economic factors than health issues. It is of interest that the first ever health treaty negotiated under the World Health Organization, the Framework Convention on Tobacco Control, became effective February 27, 2005. The United States has not ratified the treaty, despite its leadership in many areas of tobacco control, including documentation of tobacco's adverse health effects.

Sloan and colleagues (2004) analyzed the economic costs in the U.S. of smoking cigarettes. They separated those costs the tobacco smoker must bear (internal costs) from the costs to others (external costs). They concluded that, over the lifetime of a one-pack-per-day male smoker, the total cost is $220,000; for a female it is $106,000. Thus, the lifetime cost of a pack of cigarettes is about $40 per pack, of which the smoker pays $33 (internal), the smoker's family $5 (external), and society $1 (external). Their analysis takes into account the fact that smoking kills smokers and thus saves Medicare and Social Security funds.

If tobacco use were a simple volitional behavior, perhaps such an economic burden would lead more quickly to people giving it up. We now understand that tobacco dependence is so strong that smoking persists. Mark Twain once remarked on how easy it was for him to stop smoking because he had done it so many times. Only about half of the chronic daily users of tobacco are able to quit without much help. Until a substitute for tobacco that is acceptable to smokers becomes available, tobacco use surely will continue.

What are some of the new directions needed?

1. There is a need to develop a nicotine inhaler that will produce a particle size similar to that in tobacco smoke. The inhalers developed years ago used irritating propellants. Such inhalers produced effective pharmacological effects but were noxious.
2. Because tobacco smoke contains a large variety of chemicals, it is important to consider other substances besides nicotine—for example, the compounds in tobacco smoke that alter the levels of naturally occurring substances in the brain that are important in how people feel, such as monoamine oxidase (MAO; Yu and Boulton, 1987; Khalil et al., 2000; Hauptmann and Shih, 2001). Compared to nonsmokers, drug-free schizophrenic tobacco smokers have reduced whole blood or platelet MAO activity. Most

mentally ill patients smoke more than those who are normal. Could they be self-medicating with tobacco smoke? Positron emission tomography brain scan images of tobacco smokers with about 40–60 percent reduced brain/body MAO_A and MAO_B activity (Fowler et al., 1996a, 1999b) support that concept. The neurotransmitter dopamine is biotransformed to inactive metabolites by $MAO_{A,B}$. Theoretically, its inhibition would prolong the action of dopamine; however, inhibition of an enzyme by 80 percent or more is usually necessary for a pharmacological effect. Hence, the significance of $MAO_{A,B}$ inhibition in tobacco smokers is unclear. The finding that administering nicotine does not completely treat tobacco withdrawal supports the hypothesis that chemicals in smoke besides nicotine contribute to physically based dependence. Such neuroscience research addressing factors in addition to nicotine in the dependence process will open new treatment avenues in the twenty-first century. The research by George et al. (2005) using the MAO_B inhibitor selegiline is a step in this direction. In the case of MAO_A inhibitors, they must be of the reversible type; otherwise, there is possible precipitation of hypertensive crises due to tyramine containing foods (the cheese effect). Chronic tobacco smoking, however, does not precipitate the cheese effect. There is evidence that other constituents in tobacco smoke such as harmine have pharmacological effects.

Brody et al. (2004), using another brain mapping technique, magnetic resonance imaging, found that compared to nonsmokers cigarette smokers have reductions in the gray matter of some areas of the brain related to the years of smoking. The disturbing results of this preliminary study need to be replicated by others. Such findings may affect the ability of chronic tobacco smokers to quit and argues for the possibility that at least some tobacco users may require long term if not lifetime treatment to sustain tobacco abstinence.

3. Research carried out in our laboratory has concentrated on the chemical mechanisms of brain dependence and withdrawal of nicotine. If dopamine is the key neurotransmitter that nicotine releases to produce reinforcement, dopamine agonist therapies should be far more effective than they have so far proven to be. The fact that bupropion is an effective cessation treatment supports this conclusion, but limitations in its effectiveness also raise

the possibility that it does not target other important mechanisms in tobacco dependence. Which mechanisms are most important, and which medications might provide the most effective treatment remain elusive and raise many questions. For example, why isn't L-DOPA an effective cessation treatment? What about the use of selective D_1, D_2, D_3, D_4, or D_5 agonist therapies as these agents *have* become clinically available? The observation that the brain utilization of β-[^{11}C]-L-DOPA is reduced after overnight withdrawal and reversed with nicotine in nicotine-dependent monkeys (Domino et al., 2004) suggests that new treatment approaches are necessary. Is this observation in monkeys true of those tobacco smokers who have difficulty quitting smoking? How long does it take the nicotine-dependent brain to recover to normal? Inasmuch as most old brain protein is replaced by new ("brain protein turnover") within about one week to one month, the long-lasting craving for tobacco smoking probably involves primarily psychological factors. This also implies that some smokers would need long-term to life-long treatments. New treatments must address physical and chemical brain changes as well as the *pathopsychological* mechanisms of addiction. Although we enter the twenty-first century with *a* significant advance in the understanding of tobacco use and approaches to treatment, it is clear that there is yet much work to be done until all who wish to cease their tobacco use can do so.

REFERENCES

Brody, A. L., Mandelkern, M. A., Jarvik, M. E., Lee, G. S., Smith, E. C., Huang, J. C., Bota, R. G., Bartzokis, G., and London, E. D. 2004. Differences between smokers and nonsmokers in regional gray matter volumes and densities. *Biological Psychiatry* 55:77–84.

Domino, E. F., Mirzoyan, D., and Tsukada, H. 2004. N-methyl-aspartate antagonists as drug models of schizophrenia: a surprising link to tobacco smoking. *Progress in Neuro-Psychology & Biological Psychiatry* 28: 801–11.

Feldman, E. A., and Bayer, R. 2004. *Unfiltered: Conflicts over Tobacco Policy and Public Health.* Cambridge, Mass.: Harvard University Press.

Fowler, J. S., Volkow, N. D., Logan, J., Pappas, N., King, P., MacGregor, R., Shea, C., Garza, V., and Gatley, S. J. 1998. An acute dose of nicotine does not inhibit MAO B in baboon brain in vivo. *Life Sciences* 63:19–23.

Fowler, J. S., Volkow, N. D., Wang, G. H., Pappas, N., Logan, J., MacGregor, R., Alexoff, D., Shea, C., Schlyer, D., and Wolf, A. P. 1996a. Inhibition of monoamine oxidase B in the brains of smokers. *Nature* 379: 733–36.

Fowler, J. S., Volkow, N. D., Wang, G. H., Pappas, N., Logan, J., Shea, C., Alexoff, D., MacGregor, R., Schlyer, D., Zezulkova, I., and Wolf, A. P. 1996b. Brain monoamine oxidase A inhibition in cigarette smokers. *Proceedings of the National Academy of Sciences USA* 93:14065–69.

George, T. P., Vessicchio, J.C., and Weinberger, A. H. 2005. Development of selegiline for smoking cessation. Abstracts, Society for Research on Nicotine and Tobacco, p. 13. Prague, Czech Republic, March 20–23.

Hauptmann, N., and Shih, J. C. 2001. 2-Naphthylamine, a compound found in cigarette smoke, decreases both monoamine oxidase A and B catalytic activity. *Life Sciences* 68:1231–41.

Khalil, A. A., Steyn, S., and Castagnoli, N. 2000. Isolation and characterization of a monoamine oxidase inhibitor from tobacco leaves. *Chemical Research in Toxicology* 13:31–35.

Sloan, F. A., Ostermann, J., Picone, G., Canover, C., and Taylor, Jr., D. H. 2004. *The Price of Smoking.* Cambridge, Mass.: MIT Press.

Yu, P. H., and Boulton, A. A. 1987. Irreversible inhibition of monoamine oxidase by some components of cigarette smoke. *Life Sciences* 41: 675–82.

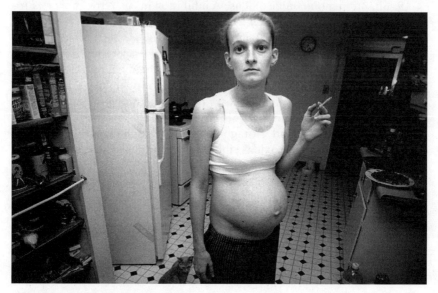

Untitled, by Brenda Ann Kenneally

9

Could Nutritional Factors Influence the Development and Maintenance of Addiction to Nicotine?

GARY A. GIOVINO, PH.D., M.S.

Major cross-sectional population studies comparing current cigarette smokers to those who have never smoked have found that cigarette smokers ("current smokers") consume fewer servings of fruits, vegetables, and whole grains, and consume more servings of caffeinated beverages, alcoholic beverages, processed meats, snack foods, fats, and oils (Wichelow et al., 1988; Subar et al., 1990; Nuttens et al., 1992; Bolton-Smith et al., 1993; Serdula et al., 1996). Current smokers are also less likely than former smokers and those who have never smoked to eat breakfast (Schoenborn and Benson, 1988). Further, Subar and colleagues (1990) and Wichelow and colleagues (1988) observed an inverse relationship between consumption of fruits, vegetables, and whole cereal grains and the number of cigarettes smoked each day. The dietary patterns of long-term former smokers (that is, persons who have been smoke-free for at least one year) are more similar to those of never smokers, whereas the diets of smokers who quit recently resemble those of current smokers (Bolton-Smith et al., 1993). The findings from these cross-sectional studies are often interpreted as indicating that smokers are less health conscious than people who do not smoke and that heavier smokers are less health conscious than lighter smokers. This interpretation makes great sense in that those who have resisted the temptation to begin smoking or relapse after they have quit are likely to place a high value on health and thus to make choices about other health-related behaviors that are consistent with their priorities.

These cross sectional studies, however, cannot be used to define the direction of relationships and thus in this case leave open the possibility that suboptimal nutrition "came first" and thereby is actually a risk factor for starting and continuing cigarette smoking. It may be that people who are well nourished are less likely to seek out the pleasures of smoking in the first place. In addition, among people who have experimented with cigarettes, those who are well nourished may be less likely to escalate than those who are more poorly nourished. Also, those who are well nourished might be less bothered by withdrawal symptoms, such as increased hunger and constipation, than are individuals with poor diets.

Animal studies indicate that caloric restriction increases the likelihood of self-administration of a variety of substances, including nicotine (Donny et al., 1998; Carr, 2002; Stuber et al., 2002). An appetite suppressant, nicotine may be especially reinforcing in such situations (Grunberg, 1992). We do not know whether restricting key nutrients other than calories also influences the likelihood of drug self-administration.

Research with animal models also indicates that simple sugars may function as alternative reinforcers and suppress self-administration of nicotine (Campbell and Carroll, 2000). In addition to increasing caloric intake, simple sugars have some effects that are similar to addictive drugs in that they stimulate production of the naturally occurring brain chemical, dopamine (dopamine elevations are produced by most addictive drugs; Colantuoni et al., 2002). West's work (2001) suggests that chewing glucose tablets could help smokers quit.

Consuming fruits and vegetables may promote satiety, both by increasing consumption of micronutrients and phytochemicals and by increasing bulk (Fuhrman, 2003; Rolls et al., 2004). Many smokers use cigarettes to stimulate bowel movements (often with coffee). The presence of adequate fiber provided by consumption of large amounts of fruits, vegetables, and whole grains, along with adequate water intake, may lower the incidence of constipation among people trying to quit smoking (Hajek et al., 2003). An anecdotal report indicates that people who were switched to a diet of primarily uncooked foods (62 percent of calories ingested) to reduce hypertension and body weight became more sensitive to cigarette smoke and alcohol. The authors report that 80 percent of study subjects who smoked or drank alcohol stopped spontaneously, although the actual number of quitters and the duration of abstinence are not reported (Douglass et al., 1985). Some study participants reported that the raw food diet facilitated long-term appetite control. Perhaps enhanced satiety also reduced the perceived need for tobacco and alcohol.

U.S. dietary guidelines and leading nutritional experts and researchers recommend a diet rich in whole cereal grains, fruits, and vegetables (Trowell and Burkitt, 1981; Ornish et al., 1998, 2005; McDougall, 1998; Esselstyn, 2001; Lemole, 2001; Willett, 2001; Nestle, 2002; Fraser, 2003; Fuhrman, 2003; Campbell and Campbell, 2004). Such a diet can lower the risk of cardiovascular disease, several cancers, diabetes, arthritis, autoimmune diseases, and obesity. The possibility that such a diet might contribute to substance abuse treatment, or even emerge as an important component of comprehensive substance abuse treatment is provocative but merits systematic exploration. Data from the National Health and Nutrition Examination Survey (NHANES) indicate that only 10.4 percent of the calories consumed by U.S. adults come from fruits, fruit juices, or vegetables (Block, 2004). Thus, fewer than 10 percent of the calories consumed by U.S. adults come from raw foods. This means that U.S. adults consume lower levels of raw foods that were concluded to be healthful in studies such as the classic 1946 study by Pottenger, who suggested the existence of a threshold of benefit for consumption of raw food on health and mortality in house cats. It would be interesting to compare nicotine and other drug self-administration in animals fed on laboratory chow with those fed isocaloric amounts of raw foods. Analogically, human drug effects and intake could be studied by designing research to include an experimental condition that mimics an "American" diet (Block, 2004), as well as conditions that substantially vary the percentage of calories from fruits, vegetables, nuts, and seeds (both cooked and uncooked). Dietary assessments administered to participants in smoking cessation studies would provide important observational data. If justified by the animal or human data, randomized intervention trials to study the effect of a whole foods, plant-based diet on nicotine self-administration would be warranted.

Among the specific research questions that might be asked are:

1. Does suboptimal nutrition increase the probability of initiating smoking?
   a. Could micronutrient deficiency (deficiencies) increase the probability of initiation?
   b. Could the composition of the diet (e.g., percent uncooked food, percent from animal sources) influence initiation?
   c. Is a poorly nourished body (brain) more susceptible to stress and thus in a state in which nicotine is more reinforcing?
   d. Could suboptimal nutrition increase behavioral problems, which are associated with increased probability of smoking initiation?
   e. Does suboptimal nutrition in utero lead to decreased cognitive functioning, school performance, and/or athletic performance—factors that are associated with cigarette smoking among young people?
   f. Do children who were breastfed have greater protection against initiating smoking—both in terms of nutrients delivered to the body and the proper development of neurological pathways?
2. Does suboptimal nutrition decrease the probability of quitting smoking?
   a. Could micronutrient deficiency (deficiencies) exacerbate withdrawal and/or decrease the probability of cessation? For example, low levels of vitamin D can contribute to mild depression, anger/irritability, anxiety, and mental dullness. Someone attempting to quit who is deficient in vitamin D (due either to inadequate intake in food or to minimal sun exposure) could have an especially difficult time with nicotine withdrawal.
   b. Does relatively greater consumption of fruits and vegetables, including relatively high percentages that are uncooked, contribute to satiety and lessen withdrawal? If so, would dietary intervention increase the probability of abstinence?
   c. Would high volume of water and fiber decrease the constipation that can accompany quitting and increase the probability of abstinence?
   d. Is a poorly nourished body (brain) more susceptible to stress and thus to relapse?

The use of tobacco is influenced by multiple factors, including personal and environmental ones, as well as the design of the product itself. Whether any nutritional variables will ever be added to the list of known etiologic factors is a question that only further research can answer, but such research is needed, for it could provide a useful tool for families seeking to prevent nicotine addiction in their children and for individuals seeking to stop using tobacco. Research of this nature might also apply to other addictive substances. Some day, weight control, cholesterol control, smoking cessation, and other behaviors or conditions may no longer be parsed out as distinct problems with distinct treatments. Instead, more generally nutritious patterns of eating may support broad health goals.

ACKNOWLEDGMENTS

Funding for this chapter was provided by the Robert Wood Johnson Foundation's Innovators Combating Substance Abuse Program, administered by the Johns Hopkins University School of Medicine. Thanks to Marina Picciotto and Lynn Kozlowski for interesting discussions on this topic.

REFERENCES

Block, G. 2004. Foods contributing to energy intake in the US: data from NHANES III and NHANES 1999–2000. *Journal of Food Composition and Analysis* 17:439–47.

Bolton-Smith, C., Woodward, M., Brown, C. A., and Tunstall-Pedoe, H. 1993. Nutrient intake by duration of ex-smoking in the Scottish Heart Health Study. *British Journal of Nutrition* 69:315–32.

Campbell, T. C., and Campbell, T. M. 2004. *The China Study: The Most Comprehensive Study of Nutrition Ever Conducted and the Startling Implications for Diet, Weight Loss, and Long-Term Health*. Dallas: Benbella Books.

Campbell, U. C., and Carroll, M. E. 2000. Acquisition of drug self-administration: environmental and pharmacological interventions. *Experimental and Clinical Pharmacology* 8:312–25.

Carr, K. D. 2002. Augmentation of drug reward by chronic food restriction: behavioral evidence and underlying mechanisms. *Physiological Behavior* 76:353–64.

Colantuoni, C., Rada, P., McCarthy, J., Patten, C., Avena, N. M., Chadeayne, A., and Hoebel, B. G. 2002. Evidence that intermittent, excessive sugar intake causes endogenous opioid dependence. *Obesity Research* 10:478–88.

Donny, E. C., Caggiula, A. R., Mielke, M. M., Jacobs, K. S., Rose, C., and Sved, A. F. 1998. Acquisition of nicotine self-administration in rats: the effects of dose, feeding schedule, and drug contingency. *Psychopharmacology* (Berlin) 136(1):83–90.

Douglass, J. M., Rasgon, I. M., Fleiss, P. M., Schmidt, R. D., Peters, S. N., and Abelmann, E. A. 1985. Effects of a raw food diet on hypertension and obesity. *Southern Medical Journal* 78:841–44.

Esselstyn, C. B., Jr. 2001. Resolving the coronary artery disease epidemic through plant-based nutrition. *Preventive Cardiology* 4:171–77.

Fraser, G. E. 2003. *Diet, Life Expectancy, and Chronic Disease: Studies of Seventh Day Adventists and Other Vegetarians.* New York: Oxford University Press.

Fuhrman, J. 2003. *Eat to Live.* Boston: Little, Brown.

Grunberg, N. E. 1992. Cigarette smoking and body weight: a personal journey through a complex field. *Health Psychology* 11:26–31.

Hajek, P., Gillison, F., and McRobbie, H. 2003. Stopping smoking can cause constipation. *Addiction* 98:1563–67.

Lemole, G. 2001. *The Healing Diet.* New York: HarperCollins.

McDougall, J. A. 1998. *The McDougall Program for a Healthy Heart.* New York: Penguin Putnam.

Nestle, M. 2002. *Food Politics. How the Food Industry Influences Nutrition and Health.* Berkeley: University of California Press.

Nuttens, M. C., Romon, M., Ruidavets, J. B., Arveiler, D., Ducimetiere, P., Lecerf, J. M., Richard, J. L., Cambou, J. P., Simon, C., and Salomez, J. L. 1992. Relationship between smoking and diet: the MONICA-France Project. *Journal of Internal Medicine* 231:349–56.

Ornish, D., Weidner, G., Fair, W. R., Marlin, R., Pettengill, E. B., Raisin, C. J., Dunn-Emke, S., Crutchfield, L., Jacobs, F. N., Barnard, R. J., Aronson, W. J., McCormac, P., McKnight, D. J., Fein, J. D., Dnistrain, A. M., Weinstein, J., Ngo, T. H., Mendell, N. R., and Carroll, P. R. 2005. Intensive lifestyle changes may affect the progression of prostate cancer. *Journal of Urology* 174:1065–70.

Ornish, D., Scherwitz, L. W., Billings, J. H., Brown, S. E., Gould, K. L., Merritt, T. A., Sparler, S., Armstrong, W. T., Ports, T. A., Kirkeeide, R. L., Hogeboom, C., and Brand, R. J. 1998. Intensive lifestyle changes for reversal of coronary heart disease. *JAMA* 280:2001–7.

Pottenger, F. 1946. The effect of heat-processed foods and metabolized vitamin D milk on the dentofacial structures of experimental animals. *American Journal of Orthodontics and Oral Surgery* 32:467–85.

Rolls, B. J., Ello-Martin, J. A., and Tohill, B. C. 2004. What can intervention studies tell us about the relationship between fruit and vegetable consumption and weight management? *Nutrition Reviews* 62:1–17.

Schoenborn, C. A., and Benson, V. 1998. Relationship between smoking and other unhealthy habits. *Advance Data from Vital and Health Statistics.* No. 154. DHHS Pub. No. (PHS) 88–1250. Hyattsville, Md.: Public Health Service.

Serdula, M. K., Byers, T., Mokdad, A. H., Simoes, E., Mendlein, J. M., and Coates, R. J. 1996. The association between fruit and vegetable intake and chronic disease risk factors. *Epidemiology* 7:161–65.

Stuber, G. D., Evans, S. B., Higgins, M. S., Pu, Y., and Figlewicz, D. P. 2002. Food restriction modulates amphetamine-conditioned place preference and nucleus accumbens dopamine release in the rat. *Synapse* 46:83–90.

Subar, A. F., Harlen, L. C., and Mattson, M. E. 1990. Food and nutrient intake differences between smokers and non-smokers in the US. *American Journal of Public Health* 80:1323–29.

Trowell, H. C., and Burkitt, D. P. 1981. *Western Diseases: Their Emergence and Prevention.* Cambridge, Mass.: Harvard University Press.

West, R. 2001. Glucose for smoking cessation: does it have a role? *CNS Drugs* 15:261–65.

Wichelow, M. J., Golding, J. F., and Treasure, F. P. 1988. Comparison of some dietary habits of smokers and non-smokers. *British Journal of Addiction* 83:295–304.

Willett, W. C. 2001. *Eat, Drink, and Be Healthy.* New York: Simon & Schuster.

II

Special Populations

10

Addiction and Pregnancy

HENDREE JONES, PH.D.

In the United States, policymakers view drug-addicted persons through two lenses. Through one lens, drug addiction is a moral failing and drug-addicted persons are criminals. Through the other, drug-addicted individuals are the suffering victims of a serious illness. As a result, the effort to stop drug use includes both prosecution and treatment, with a majority of resources focused on prosecution. Prosecution is premised on the view that drug abuse is a choice that can be influenced by threats and coercion, whereas treatment is premised on the view that drug addiction is a medical illness and separates the person from the disliked behavior.

Where pregnant women are concerned, some see the drug user as a criminal, forcing drugs on her fetus. Others define the woman as lacking control over the conditions necessary to provide adequate fetal health and see her negative behaviors as symptoms of the severity of her illness. Where some see pregnant women and their fetuses as adversaries, others see them as interdependent. On one hand, the solution to the problem of perinatal addiction is to prosecute women into submission; on the other, it is to empower them, providing the education women need to be able to make choices appropriate for a healthy pregnancy.

The purpose of this chapter, which explores the policy implications of these diverging views, is threefold: history, underlying philosophy, and unmet goals of the prosecution approach to addiction in pregnancy.

Historical Context

The concern over pregnant women using drugs in the U.S. is not new. In the 1800s, 66–75 percent of opium addicts were women and the most common drug source was medical prescriptions (Kandall, 1996). Women were considered the "weaker sex," lacking ability to cope with pain and requiring medication. During the late 1800s, physicians recognized the neonatal opioid withdrawal syndrome and the need to treat the newborns of addicted mothers with morphine to prevent morbidity and mortality (Earle, 1888).

By the 1900s, physicians were better about prescribing narcotics and legitimate drug supplies shrank. As a result, women unable to stop using drugs were forced to seek them from illegitimate sources. As the U.S. sought international power, the need to control illegal drugs increased and culminated in the passing of the Harrison Narcotic Act of 1914, which greatly changed narcotic prescribing and dispensing practices by requiring addictive substances to be prescribed by licensed health professionals. Although addiction treatment was in its infancy, some physicians treated persons addicted to morphine with prescription opioids, including morphine. This practice was prohibited in 1919 when the Supreme Court ruled that physicians could no longer prescribe narcotics for the main purpose of treating drug addiction. One consequence of this was to drive addiction treatment away from mainstream medicine.

In the 1960s and 1970s, as substance abuse became an important social issue, in part due to recognition of high rates of abuse among the young, including Vietnam veterans, advocates for women's health and social equality highlighted the special treatment needs of substance-abusing women, including pregnant women. In the 1970s, the National Institute on Drug Abuse (NIDA) funded projects that addressed addiction among women, with much of its initial effort focused on pregnant drug-using women (Kandall, 1996). For example, NIDA's "Perinatal 20" project focused on the special needs of pregnant and postpartum women using "crack" cocaine and cocaine.

During the "War on Drugs" of the 1980s, the media proclaimed a "crack baby" epidemic. Stories cast these children as damaged and unteachable and their mothers as selfish and unloving. The reports of "crack babies" fueled the most punitive strategy toward drug-using pregnant women to date: the prosecution of pregnant women under a variety of state laws involving assault with a deadly weapon, delivery of a controlled substance to a minor, and child abuse (Paltrow, 1990; Mariner et al., 1990).

Meanwhile, emergence of arguments for "fetal rights" has created the perception that mother and fetus are adversaries. It has also obscured the role of the father in the development of the child and his role in fetal health. At the same time, rapid medical advances over the past twenty years have led to increased scrutiny of pregnant women and resulted in holding mothers responsible for any fetal and neonatal problems. If a woman received inadequate prenatal care, made poor nutritional choices, or took drugs, drank alcohol, or smoked, she is held responsible for causing her fetus's or neonate's problems and therefore is considered a bad mother. Although it is understandable that many have argued for controlling a pregnant woman's behavior to protect her fetus, the result has been to transform pregnant women into criminals, punishable by law for making poor choices.

The Prosecution Approach

The prosecution approach uses the criminal justice system to curtail the use of illicit drugs during pregnancy. As one prosecutor has stated, "We are not . . . interested in . . . sending [pregnant drug users] to jail. We are just interested in getting them to stop using drugs before they do something horrible to their babies" (Lewin, 1990). Alternatively, it was argued that, if stopping drug use was truly the goal, there was no need to pass special laws specifically targeting pregnant women because each state already had laws criminalizing the manufacture, delivery, or possession of narcotics. In fact, it was argued that singling out pregnant women who take drugs for special scrutiny suggested to some that what was actually being punished was the condition of pregnancy and that a consequence might be to simply encourage pregnant women to work harder to hide their addiction, thereby reducing their likelihood of obtaining treatment and quitting drug use (Mariner et al., 1990).

It is certainly a laudable goal to stop pregnant women from actions that would harm their fetuses and increase the possibility of a poor birth outcome. It is important, however, to examine carefully what harm we are trying to prevent, what acts cause this harm, what responsibilities a pregnant woman has to prevent harm, and whether this harm can be prevented by prosecution (Mariner et al., 1990).

If what is to be prevented is *any* harm whatsoever, the source of harm is not important. Anything that causes harm should be open to prosecution: failing to get prenatal care or proper nourishment, smoking cigarettes, taking (or not taking) medications for mental disorders (when doing so has consequences for the fetus, as with depression), or ingesting one or more alcoholic drinks should all be prosecuted. This is especially important because illicit drugs are often believed to be the most harmful, yet the toxic effects of alcohol and cigarette smoking are well established and may be equally or more harmful than illicit drugs (Slotkin, 1998). In light of the evidence that drug-using fathers can contribute to congenital abnormalities (Savitz et al., 1991), it could be argued that they too should be subject to prosecution.

If the harm to be avoided is any type of physical or mental damage to the fetus, this implies that the woman must take care to prevent avoidable injury. But how would the law define what the standards are of normal pregnancy and fetal health and well-being? Would women involved in car accidents or who developed an untreated (or untreatable) disease be prosecuted for causing injury to the fetus? How would a determination of the cause of harm be made? This would be problematic as the developmental status of a child is determined by a plethora of genetic and environmental influences (Mariner et al., 1990).

If the harm to be prevented results directly from drug use, proving a cause-and-effect relationship is highly problematic. Many children are born with normal outcomes despite alcohol and/or drug exposure (see, e.g., Messinger et al., 2004; Singer et al., 2004). Women who use alcohol and drugs during pregnancy do so in the context of complex social and environmental factors, including poor nutrition, poor housing conditions, exposure to environmental toxins and diseases, stress, and depression, which can all impact postnatal outcome (Robins and Mills, 1993). Stopping drug use will not guarantee a healthy baby. In fact, low birth weight—an important predictor of later developmental delay (Cooke and Foulder-Hughes, 2003)—is more prevalent among women in jails than among the general population (17 vs. 7.6 percent; Mertens, 2001; U.S. Department of Health and Human Services, 2000).

To what lengths should society go to detect drug use by pregnant women? Criminal justice and child protective services are forcing health care workers to be informants and enforcers with drug testing of pregnant women. This creates problems with confidentiality and sets up an adversarial relationship between women and health care workers in general. In addition, how a woman's drug use is detected is critical as accurate detection of drug exposure depends on the method used. For example, a 43 percent false-positive rate for cocaine was found when drug screens were not conformed with gas chromatography/mass spectrometry. Also, some illicit drugs are harder to detect than others (Moore et al., 1995). This is especially concerning because in many states newborns can be taken from their mothers upon detection of a single drug-positive urine sample using any type of drug screen.

One of the goals of prosecuting a woman for using drugs is to deter continued use or provide an incentive for her to stop using drugs by requiring her to enter a treatment program (Mariner et al., 1990). Treatment is not always available to pregnant women, however; only 34 percent of federally funded programs have pregnancy or postpartum services (Substance Abuse and Mental Health Services Administration, 2002). The absence of child care, the lack of transportation, and disregard of such comorbidities as exposure to violence, depression, or economic independence are a few of the barriers women face in entering and engaging in treatment. Some programs claim they offer addiction treatment for women instead of incarceration; this assumes there is adequate treatment available and that the terms of treatment success or failure are clearly determined (e.g., if one positive urine test means a failed treatment attempt, most women will likely fail as relapse is a natural part of recovery).

Prosecuting pregnant women does not always protect the fetus if women will avoid prenatal care and hospital delivery when detection of drug use could lead to loss of custody and incarceration. There is no evidence that incarcerating drug-addicted women has served the goal of deterrence. Pregnant women who use drugs need help. All prosecution can accomplish is conviction and punishment.

Another stated goal of the prosecution approach is to protect the newborn child from harm. The state may take custody of the infant on the assumption that doing so protects him or her. It also is not known whether multiple foster placements is a better alternative for the child than remaining with a drug-using mother, but it appears that many mothers in treatment can function effectively (Lester et al.,

2004). Often babies reside for extended periods in the hospital as "boarder babies." For these babies also, the emotional and social deprivation they face in these environments may cause more harm than living with the mother. The paucity of resources devoted to caring for children born to drug-using women reveals the falsehood that the purpose of the separation of the child from the mother is to protect the child. Rather, it is to punish the mother for her poor choices. Prenatal drug use alone does not predict postnatal abuse or neglect. If the mother demonstrates behaviors sufficient to show abuse or neglect, existing law is adequate to take the child into custody for its own protection.

The Need for Better Policy

A number of major medical societies, including the American Academy of Pediatrics and the American Medical Association, have concluded that a prosecution approach to drug use during pregnancy is bad policy and contrary to good health care for a number of reasons:

1. Drug use is already illegal, so imposing harsher penalties for pregnant women will not increase the deterrent effect that already exists; furthermore, incarceration is more expensive than most forms of drug treatment.
2. Incarceration while pregnant can have negative consequences for fetal development because of the unhealthful conditions in jail and prison.
3. Fear of prosecution deters women from seeking treatment and care by instilling fear of punishment (either incarceration for themselves or the removal of their children).
4. The prosecution approach provides a false sense of security that prenatal drug exposure is being addressed and ignores the fact that there is a severe shortage of treatment in this country.

Prosecution of pregnant, drug-using women is based on misguided attempts to stop drug use. It fosters the illusion that society is protecting the future generation. In reality, prosecution substitutes punishment for protection and help. By treating women as adversaries to their own children, it marginalizes women and places children at risk by relegating them to an inadequate system of institutional or foster care. Making pregnancy one of the elements in a crime has frightening consequences. It adversely affects the way we think about pregnancy and women and negates the role of men in creating and raising children. The effects of drug use are harmful to women, children, and families, and adding the insult of criminal prosecution can only further harm those involved. The answer lies not in prosecution of women but in the hard work of chipping away at the underlying causes of drug abuse, providing education, access to medical care, drug treatment, and economic mechanisms to help women achieve independence. Treating drug use during pregnancy as a crime will only exacerbate the problem.

REFERENCES

Cooke, R. W., and Foulder-Hughes, L. 2003. Growth impairment in the very preterm and cognitive and motor performance at 7 years. *Archives of Disease in Childhood* 88:482–87.

Earle, F. B. 1888. Maternal opium habit and infant mortality. *Medical Standards* 111:2–4.

Kandall, S. R. 1996. *Substance and Shadow: Women and Addiction in the United States.* Cambridge, Mass.: Harvard University Press.

Lewin, T. 1990. Drug use in pregnancy: new issues for the courts. *New York Times,* February 5.

Lester, B. M., Andreozzi, L., and Appiah, L. 2004. Substance use during pregnancy: time for policy to catch up with research. *Harm Reduction Journal* 20, no. 1:1–44.

Mariner, W. K., Glantz, L. H., and Annas, G. J. 1990. Pregnancy, drugs, and the perils of prosecution. *Criminal Justice Ethics* 9:30–41.

Mertens, D. J. 2001. Pregnancy outcomes of inmates in a large county jail setting. *Public Health Nursing* 18:45–53.

Messinger, D. S., Bauer, C. R., Das, A., Seifer, R., Lester, B. M., Lagasse, L. L., Wright, L. L., Shankaran, S., Bada, H. S., Smeriglio, V. L., Langer, J. C., Beeghly, M., and Poole, W. K. 2004. The maternal lifestyle study: cognitive, motor, and behavioral outcomes of cocaine-exposed and opiate-exposed infants through three years of age. *Pediatrics* 113:1677–85.

Moore, C., Lewis, D., and Leikin, J. 1995. False-positive and false-negative rates in meconium drug testing. *Clinical Chemistry* 41:1614–16.

Paltrow, L. M. 1990. When becoming pregnant is a crime. *Criminal Justice Ethics* 9:41–47.

Robins, L., and Mills, J. L. 1993. Effects of in utero exposure to street drugs. *American Journal of Public Health* 83:1–32.

Savitz, D. A., Schwingl, P. J., and Keels, M. A. 1991. Influence of paternal age, smoking, and alcohol consumption on congenital anomalies. *Teratology* 44:429–40.

Singer, L. T., Minnes, S., Short, E., Arendt, R., Farkas, K., Lewis, B., Klein, N., Russ, S., Min, M. O., and Kirchner, H. L. 2004. Cognitive outcomes of preschool children with prenatal cocaine exposure. *JAMA* 291:2448–56.

Slotkin, T. A. 1998. Fetal nicotine or cocaine exposure: which one is worse? *Journal of Pharmacology and Experimental Therapeutics* 285:931–45.

Substance Abuse and Mental Health Services Administration. 2002. *The DASIS Report: Facilities Offering Special Programs or Services for Women.* Arlington, Va.: Office of Applied Studies. Substance Abuse and Mental Health Services Administration, U.S. Department of Health and Human Services, Synetics for Management Decisions, Inc.

U. S. Department of Health and Human Services. 2000. *Healthy People, 2010.* 2 vols. Washington, D.C.: U.S. Department of Health and Human Services.

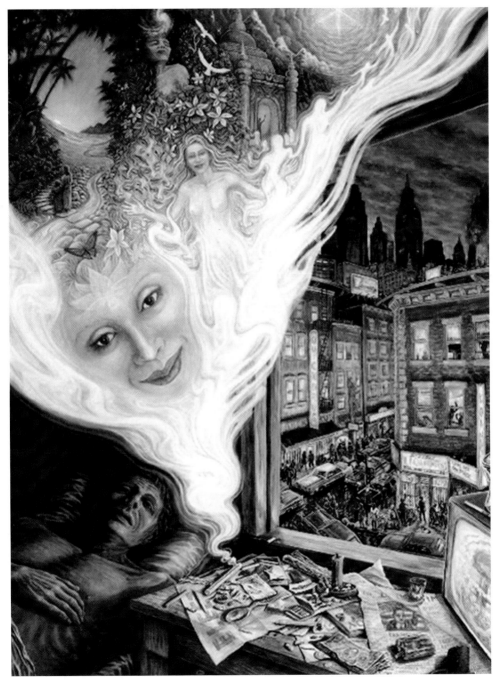

Illusion of Reality, by Mark Henson

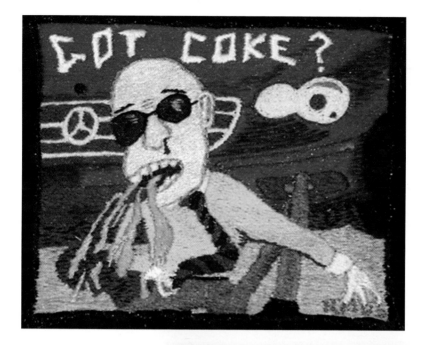

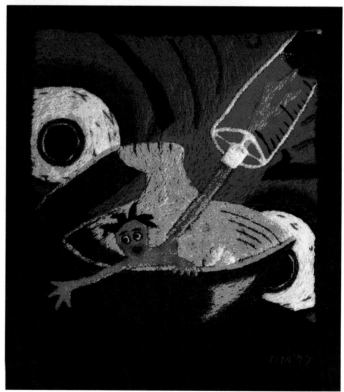

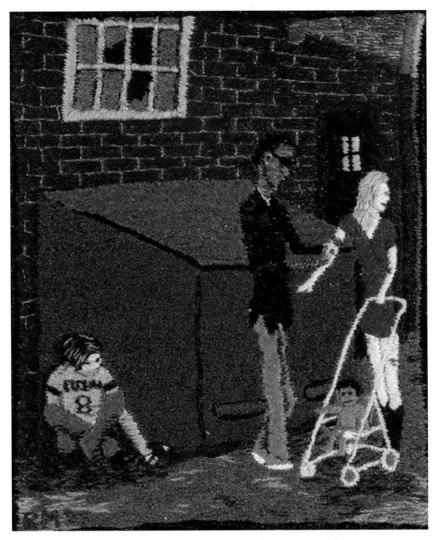

Flaco and the Prom Queen (above); *Got Coke?* (opposite, top); *Don't Get Pulled In* (opposite, bottom); all by Ray Materson

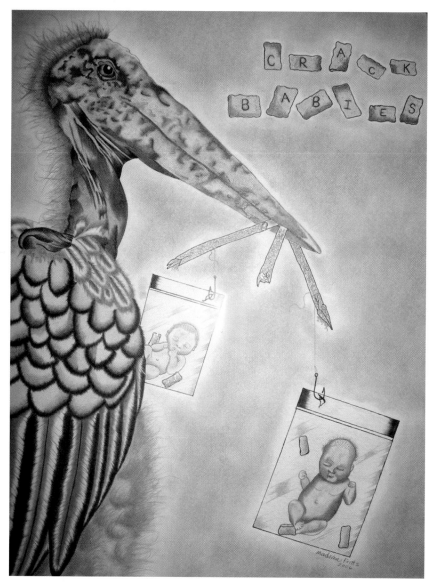

Crack Babies, by Madian Fritts

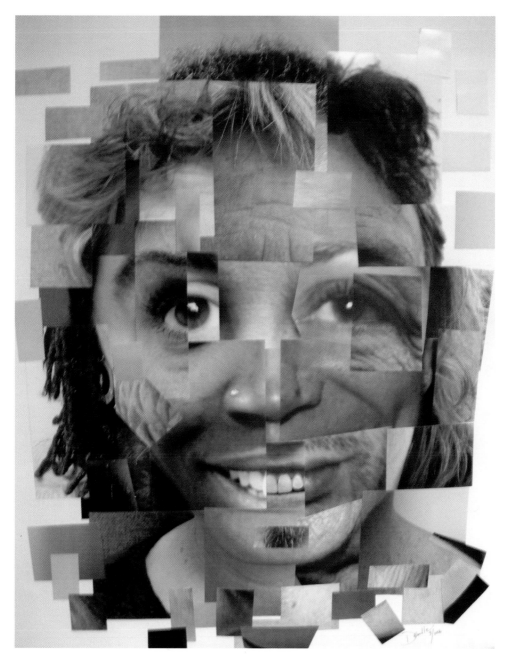

I Am the Face of Addiction and Recovery, by Denille Marion Francis

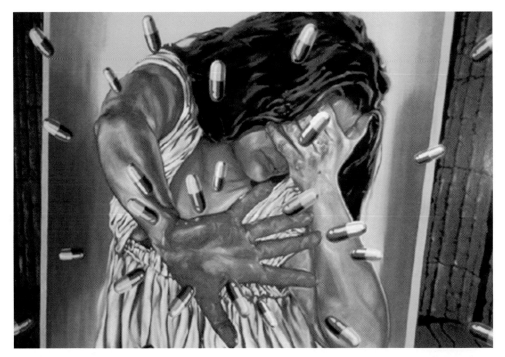

Letting Go, by Margaret Dowell

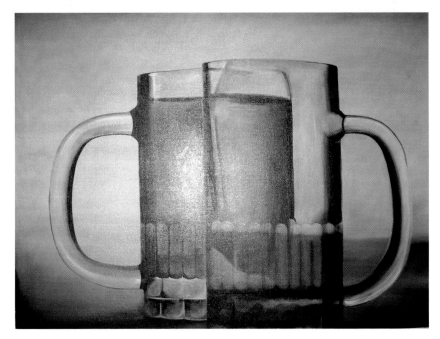

My Dear Brother, by Scott Entze

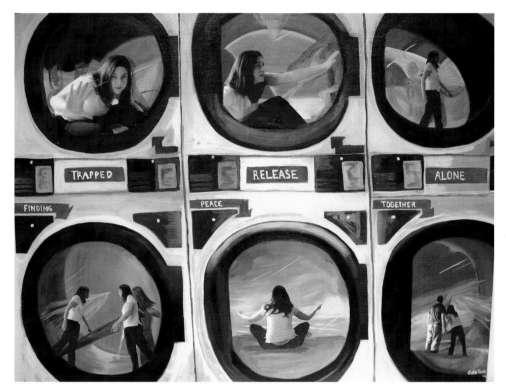

Clean: A Journey, by Julie Gross

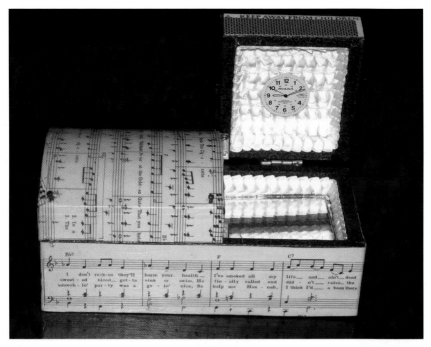

Breathlessness: A Matter of Time, by Vicki Caucutt

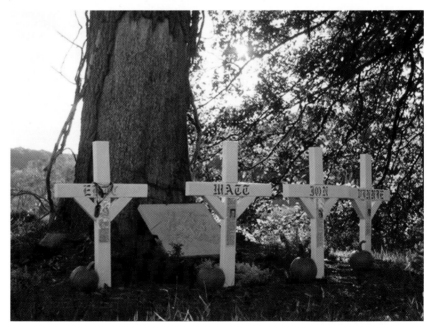

Untitled, by Laura Burns

11

Perspectives on the Risk-Benefit Ratio of Pharmacological Treatment for Adolescent Chemical Addiction

ERIC T. MOOLCHAN, M.D.

For adults with chemical dependency, recognition of the lethal and chronic nature of addiction has led to the development and approval of several widely prescribed and widely used pharmacotherapeutic agents to accompany comprehensive approaches to treatment of addiction. Prominent examples include methadone or buprenorphine for opioid addiction, naltrexone or acamprosate for alcohol addiction, and various forms of nicotine-replacement therapy or bupropion for tobacco addiction. Regulatory approvals that fuel practitioners' prescriptions and overall access to pharmacotherapies for the treatment of addictions among adults have followed conclusive evidence of safety and efficacy from empirical testing in clinical trials that do not typically include youths.

The Importance of Adolescent Substance Abuse

Despite these efforts, substance use that leads to addiction, the leading public health problem of our time, typically begins during childhood and adolescence, with many surveys continuing to show high prevalence rates for use of the various drug categories. It is safe to say that this epidemic of youth substance use and addiction will not go away anytime soon. Monitoring the Future, a survey that gathered data from twelfth graders in 128 schools throughout the nation, shows last 30-day rates of substance use ranging from 1.9 percent for hallucinogens to 48 percent for alcohol, and rates of 25 percent for cigarette smoking and 6.7 percent for use of smokeless tobacco (Johnston et al., 2005). Rates of substance use run even higher among adolescents who do not attend school. The recent National Drug Use and Health survey reveals the alarming finding that the largest increase in new or first-time users occurred among youth using opioid analgesics, among whom users increased by half a million from 2000 to 2002.

The costs of these behaviors are all too familiar. In the case of nicotine and tobacco as an example, because more than half of daily smokers eventually develop serious tobacco-related disease and die prematurely, and cessation reduces that risk (Anthonisen et al., 2005), aggressively treating tobacco use among youths not only saves years of life but also improves quality of life and has been shown to be highly cost-effective (Hall et al., 2005). Another reason to aggressively detect and address youth smoking lies in the fact that smoking is a strong predictor for use of and addiction to alcohol and other drugs (Henningfield et al., 1990; Kandel and Yamaguchi, 1993). Yet for reasons outlined below, youth tobacco addiction, along with problem alcohol use and other addictions, remains underdiagnosed and even more often undertreated.

Youth Addiction Treatment Lacks Evidence-Based Guidelines

Many adolescents want treatment for their chemical addictions and all of them deserve access to it. By the age of 17, it is estimated that half the tobacco smokers have tried to quit and failed, (U.S. Department of Health and Human Services, 1994) usually by engaging in self-generated acute abstinence methods (i.e., cold turkey) (Myers and MacPherson, 2004). The persistently high prevalence of smoking among adolescents contrasts with the lack of societal emphasis placed on helping them to quit. We can do better. Although several pharmacological adjuncts to smoking cessation have been approved for adults, the dearth of safety and efficacy data from controlled studies has limited prescribing of pharmacological agents by clinicians for adolescent smokers. Despite polls indicating adolescent smokers' desire to quit, the combination of systemic barriers to recruitment into clinical trials, high attrition and relatively low quit rates in research studies have hampered the collection of needed data, forcing practitioners to rely on guidelines based on expert opinion rather than those based on empirical findings. Considering other addictive substances, such as opioids and alcohol, for which adult pharmacotherapies are firmly established, extremely little controlled study has occurred for youths.

Legal and Ethical Barriers to Adolescent Addiction Research and Treatment

Adolescence constitutes a transitional period of sociobiological, cognitive, and emotional development between childhood and adulthood (Dahl, 2001). As "minors," adolescents are generally denied autonomy when it comes to research participation. The developmental, ethical, and legal/regulatory aspects that distinguish adolescents from adults with regard to research participation constitute one large barrier to obtaining empirical data that are needed to design and implement youth-tailored treatment regimens. Under current federal regulations, parents, not the adolescents themselves, decide whether their children will participate in research (45 CFR 46.408). Regulations also significantly restrict the kinds of research in which children, including adolescents, may participate, permitting research involving more than "minimal risk" only when there is prospect of direct benefit to individual participants or the knowledge to be gained is of "vital importance" for understanding the participant's condition or disorder (45 CFR 46.405–406). Because the federal regulations do not specifically address differences between children and adolescents, institutional review boards vary in their interpretation of the regulations. This may result in decisions that contrast with the "emancipated minor" laws in many states that allow adolescents to present for treatment for an addiction and other sensitive clinical issues on their own behalf, without an adult guardian (Santelli et al., 2003). Some of the protective mechanisms put in place because of past breaches in ethical principles of research with minors ironically now impede scientific progress that would lead to treatment benefit for young dependent users.

To make it easier for adolescent drug users to enroll in clinical trials, the concept of "mature minor" should be integrated with that level of risk. The assessment of risk should take into account not only the specific risks posed by the research itself but also the fact that adolescents may have difficulty distinguishing between scientific merit and therapeutic benefits depending on their developmental and emotional states, which might influence their decision-making capacity (Dorn et al., 1995). In establishing safeguards for research among youths, however, care must be taken not to overprotect adolescent participants by failing to recognize their autonomy.

Confidentiality is also a concern when parental permission is required, especially when research involves sensitive behaviors (such as substance use and accompanying prohibited behaviors), and may adversely influence adolescents' decisions about participation. The prospect of sensitive information being disclosed to a parent or guardian may also undermine the quality of a therapeutic alliance. This could thus potentially skew the empirical data and adversely affect a study's potential to contribute generalizable knowledge to enhance the quality and availability of treatment for youths as a segment of society. In essence, this discriminates against the youth population for the purposes of both research and, hence, evidence-based treatment.

The Philosophy of Treating Addiction in Youths

In clinical practice, decisions about treatment proceed from an assessment of the patient's current medical status, including diagnoses, prognoses, and their relative level of certainty. Diagnostic tests are of particular importance to clarify the situation and/or the patient's clinical status. In this regard, although several generations of the *Diagnostic and Statistical Manual of Mental Disorders* (DSM) criteria have been used among adults to define various drugs in research settings, these criteria have rarely been used to define nicotine or tobacco dependence in studies of these substances, and they have almost never been applied in clinical settings.

Among adolescents, the situation is even more troubling. Even for other substance categories, adaptation of the DSM criteria to adolescents is problematic. In this gray zone, confirmation of addiction or degree of addiction is especially challenging. The absence of a universally agreed-upon definition of addiction hurts the field overall in several ways (Colby, 2000; Moolchan and Mermelstein, 2002) but carries particularly serious implications for youth.

Without a universal definition, what counts as "benefit" for the patient becomes a moving (or even undefined) target. This is especially prejudicial to youth, who are seen as a "vulnerable" population that must be protected from risk, especially risk of an experimental nature.

Without a universal definition of addiction it becomes much more difficult to capture early subjective, behavioral, or physiological manifestations of addiction. In light of the use trajectory of most drugs, however, treatment approaches would be best studied among youths. The perceived vulnerability of adolescents erects an additional barrier by precluding the study of the effects of medications on the developmental trajectory of addiction as it has been argued that behaviors that have been more recently established might be easier to extinguish (Kviz et al., 1994).

Yet we must do what we can to address problem substance use among adolescents, especially when an intervention is requested. The purpose of medication within comprehensive treatment—which should typically include some form of behavioral and psychosocial support—should be explicitly established and the possibly differing agendas of the patient and the intervention team should be reconciled in some form of treatment "contract." Questions arise rather quickly here: What is it that adolescents expect from addiction treatment, particularly when they may not have suffered years of cumulative and destructive effects of their addiction or they were *required* to enter treatment (e.g., by the juvenile justice system)? How will medication fit within their overall expectation of their own efforts to heal themselves versus the efforts of others to heal them? What are the intervention team's outcome expectations or definitions of sobriety (e.g., total or relative abstinence from drug use and other compulsive behaviors, improved overall biopsychosocial health, etc.)? How proficiently can adolescents at various stages of development internalize and adopt coping skills to prevent relapse (Baumrind and Moselle, 1985; Cooper et al., 2003)? The answers to such questions provide starting points to begin shaping therapeutic goals and alliances with young patients who might be eligible for pharmacotherapies.

The Risk-Benefit Ratio in Pharmacological Interventions for Addiction in Youths

The risks involved in pharmacological interventions for addiction broadly include, obviously, medication-related adverse side effects (toxicity), as well as any medication effects on biological, cognitive, and emotional systems—specifically in the developmental context of not-yet-mature human organisms. Several theoretical and practical considerations apply to assessing the risk-benefit ratio of pharmacological treatment of addiction in adolescents. Potentially toxic side effects of medications should be weighed against the risks of the clinical course and complications of addiction, which include major disease and premature death.

"Off-label" pharmacological treatment of addicted youths should also be seen within the broader context that more than two-thirds of medications prescribed for minors have not been tested or approved for the given indication in youth. The "unapproved" use of medications is more strongly supported clinically and ethically when there is a clear "therapeutic imperative," such as an emergency or recognized life-threatening situation. With respect to addiction or compulsive use, long-term health risks of coronary heart disease, stroke, various cancers (linked to tobacco exposure), various forms of hepatitis, HIV, or drug overdose help to frame such a therapeutic need.

Finally, the risk-benefit considerations in the context of research differ somewhat from those applicable to clinical practice in that the primary benefits are the knowledge gained from the research, which accrue to science and the broader society in the short term. Adolescents as a social group benefit only indirectly or longer term. This evaluation remains difficult in situations when treatment is largely inaccessible to youths outside of research protocols.

Considerations Linked to Mechanisms of Pharmacological Treatment for Addiction

As with treatment for adult addiction, considerations of the type of medication affect the risk-benefit ratio for pharmacological treatment. Examples of such considerations would be whether the mutually agreed-upon goal is to replace (e.g., via agonist treatment) or extinguish (e.g., with an antagonist, or combined agonist/antagonist regimen) substance use and craving or to deter episodes of use with aversive therapies (e.g., disulfiram).

Several considerations should factor into decisions about agonist treatment (e.g., nicotine replacement or methadone), including toxic side effects, and the possibility of maintaining some degree of drug tolerance or potentially prolonging the clinical course of dependence. Because agonists are usually somewhat reinforcing (although less so than the original substance of abuse), safeguards are needed to assure that treatment does not perpetuate drug seeking or abuse of a substitutive medication. Treatment regimens to address recent increases in youth opioid analgesic abuse and dependence warrant particular vigilance in this respect. Conversely, few data are available to evaluate how effective *antagonist* treatment (e.g., naltrexone for opioid or alcohol addiction) is for youths, though we do know that high levels of patient motivation are typically needed for adult populations.

Beyond therapeutic use of pharmacological agents for attention deficit/hyperactive disorder (Wilens et al., 2003), little research to date has examined how pharmacological agents used to treat chemical dependence might influence neurobiological functions (affect, cognition) of development (Dahl, 2001; Wilens et al., 2003). In light of frequent perturbations of executive coping skills in dealing with stressors in young substance users, the possibility that over-reliance on pharmacotherapy might perturb the acquisition of cognitive, emotional, and behavioral coping skills essential for the long-term management of substance use disorders should be studied.

What We Should Try to Know

Important tasks lie before us for enhancing the status of the pharmacological treatment of addiction among adolescents in several domains. Regarding the interactions of adolescent development and progression of the addiction cycle, examples of outstanding questions might include: What are the long-term effects of various types of drug substitution maintenance therapy for adolescents? In nicotine addiction, for example, would reduction in cigarette consumption facilitated by nicotine replacement therapy lead to a reduction in other markers of addiction for adolescent smokers? In light of evidence that reducing smoking might facilitate eventual cessation, what balance of reduced toxin and nicotine exposure would result in reduced severity of dependence and eventual cessation success? Is there a threshold level of smoking that predicts adult dependence and eventual disease severity? How does individual sensitivity to nicotine/tobacco-related morbidity mitigate these effects? How do cognitive, emotional, and behavioral developmental factors of adolescence influence tolerability and compliance? Also, from a developmental perspective, would the use of one pharmacological agent to overcome the addiction to another perturb the development and application of therapeutic coping skills (Cooper et al., 2003)? In the face of psychiatric comorbidity among youths, how feasible is it to consider adding another medication to existing long-term polypharmacy? In this light, one of the clearest indications for a pharmacological intervention might be the failure or inadequacy of "lower-risk" behavioral treatment modalities, especially for youths who have requested treatment.

Factors that would mitigate the risks of pharmacological treatments in adolescents might include significant experience of safety and efficacy among adult populations, such as that from postmarketing data sets (e.g., nicotine-replacement therapy or bupropion for tobacco addiction). Finally, factors such as availability and cost should be considered, because adolescents have additional social and economical constraints that might limit their overall access to useful medications.

Conclusions

It is a regrettable, yet correctable, state of affairs, that because of systemic barriers and the comparatively small number of practitioners who are engaged in the treatment of youth addiction, relatively little higher-level advocacy has emerged for the aggressive treatment of adolescent addicts. Treatment professionals and others who are confronted with this epidemic must be heard by regulatory authorities so that progress can come from a concerted understanding of how to overcome an array of systemic barriers at multiple levels. At the very least, adolescents who request so should be allowed to participate on their own behalf in pharmacological research that carries the prospect of benefit, in analogy to emancipated minor laws, especially when treatment is not otherwise available. In view of the sensitive nature of addiction-related behaviors, broader use of waivers of parental permission would increase the degree of youths' participation (Moolchan and Mermelstein, 2002; Santelli and Rogers, 2002). An underlying condition for progress in the overall treatment of addiction is to view youth as a priority population that has its own perspectives, and on whose adequate treatment rests the destiny of our societal precepts of healing for addiction.

Rather than strict rules, there can only be guidelines for evaluating the risks and benefits of pharmacological treatment of addiction in youth. Despite the ultimate goal of attaining long-term or permanent abstinence from substance use, respect for youths' ongoing development, along with a myriad of yet-to-be-answered scientific and clinical questions, suggests that we reframe both rather rigid treatment approaches and endpoints. There are circumstances in which adolescents' requests for help should prompt pharmacologically facilitated reduction of subjective or objective effects of withdrawal to improve overall function, rather than immediate total abstinence. The inherent risks of any medication should be weighed against the prospect of a life caught up in the throes of insufficiently treated neurobiological imbalance due to addiction. Enhancing the yield of pharmacological treatment for adolescent chemical dependence starts with adopting more flexible research paradigms that enhance youth participation and provide solutions to challenges of translating research into clinical practice through improved policies and practice.

REFERENCES

Anthonisen, N. R., Skeans, M. A., Wise, R. A., Manfreda, J., Kanner, R. E., Connett, J. E., Lung Health Study Research Group. 2005. The effects of a smoking cessation intervention on 14.5-year mortality: a randomized clinical trial. *Annals of Internal Medicine* 15 (142):233–39.

Baumrind, D., and Moselle, K. A. 1985. A development perspective on adolescent drug abuse. *Advances in Alcohol and Substance Abuse* 4:41–67.

Colby, S. M., Tiffany, S. T., Shiffman, S., and Niaura, R. S. 2000. Measuring nicotine dependence among youth: a review of available approaches and instruments. *Drug and Alcohol Dependence* May 1; 59 (Suppl. 1): S23–39.

Cooper, M. L., Wood, P. K., Orcutt, H. K., and Albino, A. 2003. Personality and the predisposition to engage in risky or problem behaviors during adolescence. *Journal of Personality and Social Psychology* 84: 390–410.

Dahl, R. E. 2001 Affect regulation, brain development, and behavioral/emotional health in adolescence. *CNS Spectrums* 6:60–72.

Dorn, L. D., Susman, E. J., and Fletcher, J. C. 1995. Informed consent in children and adolescents: age, maturation and psychological state. *Journal of Adolescent Health* 16:185–90.

Hall, S. M., Lightwood, J. M., Humfleet, G. L., Bostrom, A., Reus, V. I., and Munoz, R. 2005. Cost-effectiveness of bupropion, nortriptyline, and psychological intervention in smoking cessation. *Journal of Behavioral Health Services and Research* 32:381–92.

Henningfield, J. E., Clayton, R., and Pollin, W. 1990. Involvement of tobacco in alcoholism and illicit drug use. *British Journal of Addiction* 85:279–91.

Johnston, L. D., O'Malley, P. M., Bachman, J. G., and Schulenberg, J. E.

2005. *Monitoring the Future National Results on Adolescent Drug Use: Overview of Key Findings, 2004.* NIH publication no. 05–5726. Bethesda, Md.: National Institute on Drug Abuse.

Kandel, D., and Yamaguchi, K. 1993. From beer to crack: developmental patterns of drug involvement. *American Journal of Public Health* 83:851–55.

Klein, J. D., Levine, L. J., and Allan, M. J. 2001. Delivery of smoking prevention and cessation services to adolescents. *Archives of Pediatric and Adolescent Medicine* 155:597–602.

Kviz, F., Clark, M., Crittenden, K., Freels, S., and Warnecke, R. 1994. Age and readiness to quit smoking. *Preventive Medicine* 23:211–22.

Moolchan, E. T., and Mermelstein, R. 2002. Research on tobacco use among teenagers: ethical challenges. *Journal of Adolescent Health* 30:409–17.

Moolchan, E. T., Radzius, A., Epstein, D., Gorelick, D., Uhl, G., Cadet, J., and Henningfield, J. 2002. The Fagerström Test of Nicotine Dependence and the Diagnostic Interview Schedule: do they diagnose the same smokers? *Addictive Behaviors* 27:101–13.

Myers, M. G., and MacPherson, L. 2004. Smoking cessation efforts among substance abusing adolescents. *Drug and Alcohol Dependence* 7 (73): 209–13.

Protection of Human Subjects. Title 45 CFR, Part 46, Code of Federal Regulations (revised June 18, 1991).

Santelli, J., and Rogers, A. S. 2002. Parental permission, passive consent, and "children" in research. *Journal of Adolescent Health* 30:409–17.

Santelli, J. S., Smith Rogers, A., Rosenfeld, W. D., DuRant, R. H., Dubler, N., Morreale, M., English, A., Lyss, S., Wimberly,, Y., Schissel, A., and the Society for Adolescent Medicine. 2003. Guidelines for adolescent health research: a position paper of the Society for Adolescent Medicine. *Journal of Adolescent Health* 33:396–409.

U.S. Department of Health and Human Services. 1994. *Preventing Tobacco Use among Young People: A Report of the Surgeon General.* Washington, D.C.: Government Printing Office.

Wilens, T. E., Faraone, S. V., Biederman, J., and Gunawardene, S. 2003. Does stimulant therapy of attention-deficit/hyperactivity disorder beget later substance abuse? A meta-analytic review of the literature. *Pediatrics* 111:179–85.

12

The Inhibitory Effect of Insurance Statutes on the Provision of Alcohol Screening and Intervention Services in Trauma Centers

LARRY M. GENTILELLO, M.D.

Each year there are more than 300,000 deaths as a result of traumatic injuries, and more than 3 million people sustain an injury requiring admission to the hospital. Because of the relatively young age of most trauma patients, more years of potential life are lost each year to injuries than to the next three leading causes of death—heart disease, cancer, and stroke—combined (National Center for Injury Prevention and Control, 2002).

For as long as trauma centers have been in existence, trauma surgeons have known that alcohol use is by far the leading risk factor for injury. Between 40 and 50 percent of patients admitted to a trauma center are under the influence of alcohol. Alcohol problems are so common in trauma center patients that 25 percent of those who do not have any alcohol in their blood at the time of admission have a positive result on a standard alcohol-screening questionnaire such as the CAGE ("Cut Down, Annoyed, Guilty, Eye Opener") or MAST (Michigan Alcohol Screening Test); this is nearly three times higher than the screen positive rate for the U.S. population at large (Rivara et al., 1993).

During the past 20 years there has been a sustained effort to increase the proportion of primary care physicians who screen their patients for an alcohol disorder. In light of the extraordinarily high prevalence of alcohol problems in trauma center patients, however, broadening the emphasis on screening to include trauma center patients should be a key next step in mainstreaming alcohol screening and interventions into medical settings.

Trauma centers are for several reasons uniquely positioned to implement screening and brief intervention programs. In other medical settings, the prevalence of alcohol-related problems is much less, so more time and resources are spent on screening than on providing actual interventions. In contrast, one of every two or three trauma patients is a potential candidate for a brief intervention, so most of the resources go toward actually providing interventions to patients who might benefit instead of toward finding cases.

Further, in most regions of the United States, all severely injured patients are triaged to a regional trauma center. A trauma center must guarantee immediate availability of a wide range of specialized staff, including trauma surgeons, orthopedists, neurosurgeons, anesthesiologists, specially trained nurses, and immediate 24-hour availability of an operating room, intensive care unit, and life-support equipment. Trauma centers must undergo a rigorous verification process, including a site visit, and demonstrate that they meet the specialty availability, equipment, facilities, and range of service criteria required by the American College of Surgeons Committee on Trauma.

This tight oversight and organizational structure provides a ready means of incorporating alcohol screening and interventions into trauma care. The Committee on Trauma of the American College of Surgeons now requires Level 1 trauma centers to provide alcohol screening and interventions, and most of our nation's Level 1 centers will provide the service to maintain their status. In comparison, incorporation of screening and interventions into primary care will require a voluntary change in the practice patterns of thousands of physicians, which has been colloquially compared to attempting to transport frogs across the room in a wheelbarrow.

A fundamental concept is that providing screening and intervention services through a trauma center can greatly simplify the process of getting services to the patients most likely to need them. A typical metropolitan region may have several hundred primary care physicians but only one or two trauma centers. Most patients with a substance use disorder also do not have a primary care physician, and, even if they did, the type of medical problem most likely to require medical attention in a problem drinker is an injury. Finally, trauma surgeons already overwhelmingly support alcohol screening and intervention services as a part of trauma care. A recent nationwide survey found that 83 percent of trauma surgeons believe it is important to talk to patients about their alcohol use and that a trauma center is an appropriate place to address alcohol problems.

Do Alcohol Screening and Intervention Work in Trauma Centers?

Clinical studies demonstrate significant reductions in alcohol intake and injury recidivism in patients who receive a brief intervention shortly after injury (Figure 12.1; Gentilello et al., 1999). People often change their behavior as a result of a crisis. For example, patients often quit smoking after having a myocardial infarction or other significant, smoking-related consequence. In a trauma center, the goal of the intervention is to capitalize on the crisis of the recent life-threatening injury to increase the patient's motivation to change and help the patient explore options for self-change or treatment-assisted change.

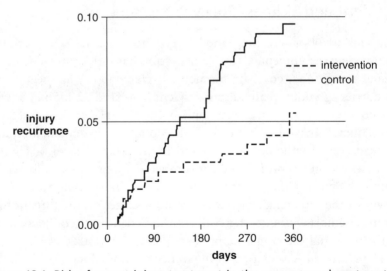

Figure 12.1. Risk of repeat injury treatment in the emergency department or admission to the trauma center in intervention and control group patients
Source: Gentilello LM, Rivara FP, Donovan DM, et al. 1999. Alcohol interventions in a trauma center as a means of reducing the risk of injury recurrence. *Annals of Surgery* 230:473–83.

One prospective, randomized trial documented a reduction by nearly 50 percent in the risk of reinjury requiring a return visit to the emergency department or admission to a trauma center (Gentilello et al., 1999). Another study documented a similar benefit to interventions in injured adolescents (Monti et al., 1999). A cost-benefit analysis documented that implementing an alcohol screening and intervention program in a trauma center or emergency department results in a significant reduction in future medical costs, with a savings of $3.81 for every dollar invested in the program (Gentilello et al., 2005a). If alcohol screening and intervention were routinely provided in trauma centers and emergency departments, the potential savings to the health care system would exceed $1.82 billion annually. This includes only direct medical costs and does not include other costs, such as lost wages, pain and suffering, rehabilitation, and costs of long-term care. For these reasons, a number of expert, consensus, and federal panels now recommend routine alcohol screening and intervention programs in trauma centers.

The Impact of the Uniform Individual Accident and Sickness Policy Provision Law

Although alcohol screening and intervention in trauma centers has been widely recommended, implementation has not been widespread. Denial of insurance coverage for alcohol-related injury has been a major barrier to widespread adoption (Gentilello et al., 2005b).

Under what is known as the Uniform Individual Accident and Sickness Policy Provision Law (UPPL), if alcohol use is documented in a medical record either by a measured blood alcohol level or clinical documentation of intoxication, insurance companies are allowed to deny payment for the patient's medical care. In a recent nationwide survey of the screening practices of trauma surgeons, the threat of insurance denials was a greater concern than cost, time, confidentiality, or the potential for offending patients (Schermer et al., 2003).

The National Association of Insurance Commissioners (NAIC) is a meeting of state insurance commissioners that provides a forum for the development of uniform policy by the development of "model laws." Drafted as a model law in 1947 by NAIC, the UPPL permits the exclusion of insurance coverage for injuries sustained by insured persons if they are found to be under the influence of alcohol or drugs:

Intoxicants and Narcotics: The insurer shall not be liable for any loss sustained or contracted in consequence of the insured's being intoxicated or under the influence of any narcotic unless administered on the advice of a physician. (National Association of Insurance Commissioners, 1947)

The UPPL was adopted as policy by 38 states, and provisionally by 4 others (e.g., narcotics only). Currently, 32 states allow denials on the basis of intoxication (Figure 12.2).

The UPPL may have been intended to reduce insurance costs by excluding alcohol-related injuries, but it has not had that effect because it is easy to circumvent. Trauma surgeons simply avoid screening patients for alcohol in jurisdictions where the UPPL is enforced. Less than 5 percent of drunk drivers injured in a crash who are taken to a

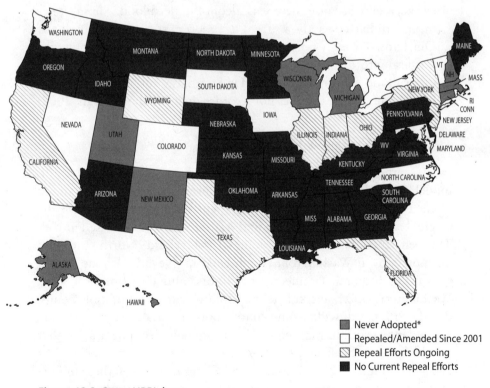

Figure 12.2. State UPPL laws
Source: Ensuring Solutions, accessed at www.ensuringsolutions.org/alcoholexclusions/

trauma center are ever convicted for "driving under the influence." Police officers do not have the time or the resources to follow every ambulance to the ER in order to obtain an evidentiary blood alcohol test. That means that, in almost every case, if the doctor does not document alcohol use at the time of injury, it is not likely to be documented by anyone else. Trauma centers that have been financially penalized by asking a patient about his or her alcohol use usually decide that it is better not to obtain this information. As a result, insurers wind up paying for most alcohol-related injuries. At the same time, however, the opportunity to provide counseling at this opportune moment is lost.

The inhibitory effect of the UPPL was highlighted in a recent article in the *Wall Street Journal* (names and locations were changed):

> Mrs. Jones, a 44-year-old waitress who lives in Baton Rouge, LA, suffered a ruptured duodenum and other internal injuries in a 1997 car accident. Because there was alcohol in her blood, she says, her insurer didn't cover the nearly $200,000 cost of her treatment at Our Lady of Mercy hospital. She filed for personal bankruptcy; the hospital wrote off the costs. The lesson? "Given the option, I don't order blood-alcohol tests," says Dr. Smith, the surgeon who treated her. "And I ask the ER docs not to order them." (Zimmerman, 2003)

The Need for Policy Change

In 2001 the NAIC unanimously approved a revision of the UPPL model. The new model law prevents insurers from denying payment of medical claims on the basis of patient intoxication. As with the original model, it is up to individual states to adopt the revised model. Thirteen states have recently done so (Maryland, North Carolina, Vermont, Iowa, Washington, North Dakota, Nevada, Rhode Island, Colorado, Indiana, Connecticut, Illinois, and Oregon, as well as Washington, D.C.), and others may follow suit. Adoption of the updated UPPL nationwide would enable more trauma centers to provide alcohol interventions that reduce the risk of recurrent injuries and that would benefit the lives of patients, their families, and society. As implied by Figure 12.2, although some states have taken these important first steps, many more have yet to act to make this important area of addiction control universal.

REFERENCES

Gentilello, L. M., Rivara, F. P., Donovan, D. M., Jurkovich, G. J., Daranciang, E., Dunn, C. W., Villaveces, A., Copass, M., and Ries, R. R. 1999. Alcohol interventions in a trauma center as a means of reducing the risk of injury recurrence. *Annals of Surgery* 230:473–83.

Gentilello, L. M., Ebel, B. E., Wickizer, T. M., Salkever, D. S., and Rivara, F P. 2005a. Alcohol interventions for trauma patients treated in emergency departments and hospitals: a cost-benefit analysis. *Annals of Surgery* 241 (4):541–50.

Gentilello, L. M., Donato, A., Nolan, S., Mackin, R. E., Liebich, F., Hoyt, D. B., and LaBrie, R. A. 2005b. Effect of the uniform accident and sickness policy provision law on alcohol screening and intervention in trauma centers. *Journal of Trauma* 59:624–31.

Monti, P. M., Colby, S. M., Barnett, N. P., Spirito, A., Rohsenow, D. J., Myers, M., Woolard, R., and Lewander, W. 1999. Brief intervention for harm reduction with alcohol-positive older adolescents in a hospital emergency department. *Journal of Consulting and Clinical Psychology* 67:989–94.

National Association of Insurance Commissioners. 2004. NAIC Model Laws, Regulations, and Guidelines. Model Regulation Service, Kansas City, Mo. Uniform Individual Accident and Sickness Policy Provision Law, II-180–1.

National Center for Injury Prevention and Control. 2002. WISQARSTM (Web-based Injury Statistics Query and Reporting System). Centers for Disease Control and Prevention. November 7. www.cdc.gov/ncipc/wisqars/.

Rivara, F. P., Jurkovich, G. J., Gurney, J. G., Seguin, D., Fligner C. L., Ries, R., Raisys, V. A., and Copass, M. 1993. The magnitude of acute and chronic alcohol abuse in trauma patients. *Archives of Surgery* 128:907–13.

Schermer, C. R., Gentilello, L. M., Hoyt, D. B., Moore, E. E., Moore, J. B., Rozycki, G. S., and Feliciano, D. V. 2003. National survey of trauma surgeons' use of alcohol screening and brief intervention. Journal of Trauma 55 (5):849–56.

Zimmerman, R. 2003. Why emergency rooms rarely test trauma patients for alcohol, drugs. *Wall Street Journal,* February 26.

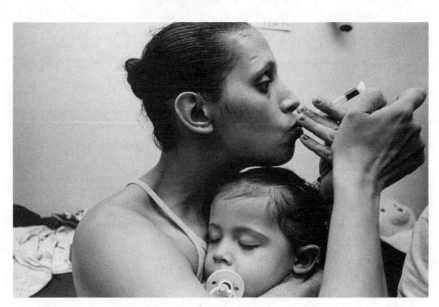

"Madonna and Child," by Brenda Ann Kenneally

13

Addiction and Multiple Morbidities in HIV-Positive Patients

HEIDI E. HUTTON, PH.D.,
PATRICIA B. SANTORA, PH.D., AND
JEFFREY J. WEISS, PH.D.

Early treatment of human immunodeficiency virus (HIV) during the 1980s focused on the individuals who contracted the disease and its complications that claimed their lives. When protease inhibitors and highly active antiretroviral therapy (HAART) became available in 1996, however, HIV was transformed from a fatal disease to a chronic one. HIV treatment consequently expanded to targeted prevention strategies, disease management, and treatment adherence.

"Triple diagnosis"—coined to describe the comorbidity of HIV infection in patients with both an addiction (to alcohol, tobacco, and/or illegal drugs) and a major psychiatric disorder—no longer adequately describes the medical state of these patients (Douaihy et al., 2003). They typically live with *multiple* morbidities, including complications from HIV infection, diseases and conditions that are side effects of prescribed medications for HIV infection, addiction, psychiatric disorders, and non-HIV-related diseases occurring in an aging HIV-positive population.

Addiction is one of the most significant barriers to the treatment of HIV-positive individuals with multiple morbidities. Whether the system of care for HIV-positive patients is medical, psychiatric, or psychosocial, addiction can compromise their access to care and their adherence to treatment plans. Addiction must be addressed if the extensive treatment needs of HIV-positive patients living with multiple morbidities are to be successfully met.

Current Challenges in the Treatment of HIV

Multiple Morbidities

Multiple medical diseases and conditions are emerging in HIV-positive individuals as their lives are prolonged because of HAART (Kilbourne et al., 2001). In 2005 an estimated 15 percent (n = 135,000) of HIV-positive individuals in the United States were more than 50 years old. This percentage is expected to increase and with it a higher incidence of complicated, multiple morbidities in these individuals. Although opportunistic infections identified with HIV will still be diagnosed, conditions *comorbid* with HIV (e.g., hepatitis C, renal disease, peripheral neuropathy, or cancer) or associated with HAART (e.g., hyperlipidemia, cardiovascular disease, or diabetes) will be more prevalent among patients receiving HIV treatment in outpatient clinics. Furthermore, as the HIV-positive population continues to age, age-related medical conditions (e.g., heart disease, cancer, cerebrovascular disease, Alzheimer disease, osteoarthritis, osteoporosis) will also emerge in these patients.

Limited knowledge exists about the incidence, severity, and health outcomes of HIV-positive individuals with multiple morbidities. Clear distinctions have not been made between epidemiological comorbidity (illnesses caused by HIV), clinical comorbidity (illnesses complicated or adversely affecting the prognosis of HIV), and co-occurring, age-related illnesses. Most of the multiple morbidities identified in HIV-positive individuals are based on prevalence but have not been stratified by age to determine their development and course in HIV disease. The potential of multiple morbidities to increase the risk for developing new illnesses or aggravating pre-existing ones is not well known. Disease management is further complicated because prevention and treatment protocols are not well established. The timing of treatment, effects of medications on comorbid diseases, and drug interactions are still being documented in case studies and controlled clinical trials.

Addiction to Alcohol, Tobacco, and/or Illegal Drugs

Addiction to alcohol, tobacco, and/or illegal drugs is one of the greatest challenges in treating HIV-positive individuals with multiple morbidities. It is the most common psychiatric disorder in HIV-positive patients, with prevalence rates as high as 40 percent. Furthermore, more than 75 percent of HIV-positive individuals with other psychiatric disorders are also addicted to legal or illegal drugs. These individuals have much poorer health than HIV-positive individuals without addictions. More specifically, HIV-positive individuals with addictions have a greater risk of developing addiction-related diseases, such as chronic lower respiratory disease, heart disease, cancer, and stroke. In addition, research indicates that addiction has been associated with more rapid disease progression and mortality in HIV. From a clinical perspective, addiction is one of the most significant barriers to HIV treatment because it compromises the individual's access to medical care and adherence to effective HIV medications.

Access to Medical Care

Addiction to alcohol and/or drugs is associated with limited access to and/or use of medical care. HIV-positive individuals who abuse alcohol and/or drugs typically seek treatment at later stages of their HIV infection when they are in overall poorer health. Further, they typically receive treatment for HIV, other medical and psychiatric disorders, and addiction, generally from multiple providers through numerous appointments at multiple sites. These individuals also often have complicated psychosocial histories involving poverty, homelessness, unemployment, violence, discrimination, and stigmatization, as well as psychiatric disorders and legal problems. Thus, the sickest, most vulnerable patients are required to navigate a complicated treatment maze, a demanding expectation for any patient, let alone the sickest of the sick.

Adherence to HAART Treatment

Addiction is also a risk factor for suboptimal adherence to HAART treatment, which directly affects the progression of the disease. Nonadherence to HAART in HIV disease can adversely affect prognosis more than nonadherence in other disease contexts because, with HAART, even very high, but less than perfect, levels of adherence can result in developing resistance to antiretroviral medication (HIV/AIDS Treatment Adherence, 2004). When HIV-positive intravenous drug users (IVDUs) and seropositive non-IVDUs have equal access to HIV treatment, IVDUs receive less benefit from HAART, as evidenced by incident increases in AIDS-defining illnesses.

Optimal Treatment Plan

Optimal treatment of HIV-positive patients with addiction and multiple morbidities requires a treatment plan that integrates substance abuse treatment and HAART at *one* medical care facility, simultaneously reducing barriers to treatment for their addiction and increasing their access to other needed medical care.

Treatment of Addiction

HIV-positive individuals who abuse drugs and/or alcohol are more difficult to treat when compared to nonaddicted HIV-positive patients. Addiction can be the critical factor that distinguishes patients' and medical providers' understandings of treatment goals. Patients often seek treatment for the multiple morbidities caused by addiction(s); they do not seek treatment for addiction. Some patients who are actively using legal or illegal drugs appear oblivious to the dangers of delaying HAART or are more concerned with less-threatening medical conditions or other life circumstances. Other patients ask their medical provider to begin HAART despite their ongoing use of legal or illegal drugs.

For providers, the goal is quite different: they want their patients to *stop using all drugs*. Addiction treatment is associated with improved rates of HAART adherence and lowered rates of utilizing hospital emergency departments compared to those not receiving addiction treatment. Medical providers often care for HIV-positive patients who are actively using or are poorly engaged in addiction treatment. Knowing that drug addiction is dangerous in itself and that it interferes with adherence to HIV treatment regimens—and to keeping medical appointments—providers face a strategic choice in working with addicted HIV-positive patients. They can advise patients to complete addiction treatment before initiating HAART—realizing that total sobriety may not be a realistic goal—or they can risk initiating HAART (to slow AIDS progression) in the belief that improved HIV outcomes would be an incentive for these patients to seek addiction treatment. For addicted patients, providers must calculate their unique risks of

HAART initiation and the possibility of developing resistance against the risks of withholding HAART.

Access to Medical Care

The organization of medical care is itself a barrier to treatment for addicted HIV-positive individuals. It is unrealistic to expect these patients to succeed in navigating a complex system of multisite and multiprovider care. Integrated, on-site medical care provided by primary clinicians would make access to care easier, especially for the sickest patients. Organizing care in this way offers the opportunity to develop a holistic health approach for HIV-positive patients, including one that facilitates quality-of-life considerations in making treatment decisions. Targeting individuals, not their diseases, creates more opportunities for patients and their providers to discuss personal health issues.

Clinical research has demonstrated that patients who regularly see the same health care *provider* are more likely to trust providers and share their concerns about other stigmatized, unhealthy behaviors, such as addiction. Similarly, HIV-positive individuals who receive their medical care and addiction treatment at the same *site* have better health outcomes and are less likely to be hospitalized compared to similar patients who receive their medical care at numerous geographic locations (Stoff et al., 2004).

Adherence to Treatment

Standard medical care often involves patient education about the risks of not treating disease or inadequate adherence to a treatment plan. For an addicted HIV-positive patient with multiple morbidities and difficult life circumstances, a treatment plan that emphasizes negative consequences in the future can be a meaningless and futile motivator. Exhortations to take medicines, keep appointments, lose weight, or monitor blood pressure to avoid yet another set of dire circumstances do not have much salience for these patients. Instead, treatment must be structured with a "rewards" strategy that emphasizes positive consequences that can occur with sobriety. Identifying rewards that are tangible and desirable to the patient, such as the ability to obtain housing or maintain friendships or employment, is more likely to motivate behavioral change and adherence to treatment plans.

Eliciting patients' priorities can help providers develop more realistic treatment plans that address multiple morbidities in ways that are sensitive to patients' life circumstances. Identifying and incorporating the patient's priorities in the treatment plan will improve communication and adherence to treatment, and thus improve health outcomes. Adapting motivational interviewing, a technique used successfully with substance abusing and addicted patients, can provide a tool for primary care providers to assess the readiness of HIV-positive patients to initiate treatment and identify the patient's priorities for treatment of multiple diseases/conditions. Motivational interviewing specifically identifies patients' ambivalence or lack of resolve in addressing medical diseases/conditions and allows them to reflect on their responsibility and commitment to improve their health. Combined with the provider's assessment of illness severity and available treatment options, motivational interviewing can help providers design and patients adhere to realistic, effective treatment plans.

Conclusion

The transformation of HIV from a fatal disease to a chronic one has created a unique set of medical, psychiatric, and psychosocial challenges in treating aging, HIV-positive individuals with multiple morbidities. Addiction, one of the most significant barriers to treating these individuals, must be addressed if the extensive treatment needs of these patients are to be successfully met. Greater attention must be paid to developing coordinated, single-site programs of care that integrate addiction treatment with care for the multiple health care needs of addicted, HIV-positive patients. To assure optimal health outcomes, an important component of such care would be to identify each patient's readiness and priorities for treatment.

REFERENCES

Douaihy, A. B., Jou, R. J., Gorske, T., and Salloum, I. M. 2003. Triple diagnosis: dual diagnosis and HIV disease. Part I. *AIDS Reader* 13:331–41.

HIV/AIDS Treatment Adherence, Health Outcomes and Cost Study Group. 2004. HIV/AIDS Treatment Adherence, Health Outcomes and Cost Study: conceptual foundations and overview. *AIDS Care* 16 (Suppl. 1):S6–21.

Kilbourne, A. M., Justice, A. C., Rabeneck, L., Rodriguez-Barrada, M., Weissman, S., for the VACS 3 Project Team. 2001. General medical and psychiatric comorbidity among HIV-infected veterans in the post-HAART era. *Journal of Clinical Epidemiology* 54 (Suppl. 1):S22–28.

Stoff, D. M., Mitnick, L., and Kalichman, S. 2004. Research issues in the multiple diagnoses of HIV/AIDS, mental illness, and substance abuse. *AIDS Care* 16 (Suppl. 1):S1–5.

14

Providing Access to Treatment for Opioid Addiction in Jails and Prisons in the United States

MARK W. PARRINO, M.P.A.

The National Institutes of Health convened a consensus development panel in 1997, "Effective Medical Treatment of Opiate Addiction," which issued a statement indicating that addiction to opioids is not a matter of will power but a medical, brain-related disorder that should be treated like any other disease. The statement held: "For decades, opioid dependence was viewed as a problem of motivation, willpower, or strength of character. Through careful study of its natural history and through research at the genetic, molecular, neuronal, and epidemiological levels, it has been proven that opiate addiction is a medical disorder characterized by predictable signs and symptoms" (National Institutes of Health, 1997).

It has been scientifically established that opioid addiction can be effectively treated through a number of interventions, including the use of maintenance pharmacotherapy using methadone and buprenorphine. Methadone has been used to effectively treat opioid addiction in the United States for the past 40 years and buprenorphine was recently approved by the Food and Drug Administration for use in treating opioid addiction as well.

It has also been well documented that addiction to drugs in general and to heroin in particular carries an enormous social stigma. This stigma is all encompassing and affects society's view of any individual who uses, misuses, and becomes addicted to opioids. In spite of proven and replicable scientific research to support the fact that opioid addiction is a medical disorder and is treatable, the stigma that surrounds addiction has interfered in providing access to care both for the general public and for incarcerated individuals.

In a recent survey of U.S. jails, Fiscella and associates examined how inmates who had been enrolled in methadone maintenance programs at the time of incarceration gained access to continued care following incarceration (Fiscella et al., 2004). They found that "very few jails elected to continue methadone following arrest." This study collected information from 246 jails and found that analgesics were routinely used to treat opioid withdrawal in 133 of the jails. Clonidine was routinely used to treat opioid withdrawal in 127 of the jails while methadone was used in 33 jails during the inmates' period of incarceration. These findings indicated "the need for the establishment of national standards for management of arrestees/inmates in methadone programs in U.S. jails as well as the need to provide improved education to help professionals working in correctional facilities regarding appropriate management of persons enrolled in methadone programs" (Fiscella et al., 2004).

In view of the fact that opioid addiction has been found to be a treatable medical disease, one might question why so few jails in the U.S. provide access to such medications for opioid-addicted inmates. The stigma already alluded to has had an overwhelming effect that has subverted the implementation of sound public policy responses to resolve clearly understood problems.

Based on their 2004 survey of corrections staff perspectives on methadone maintenance therapy in a large Southwestern jail, McMillan and associates concluded that "negative attitudes toward methadone maintenance treatment appear to be related to negative judgments about the clients the program serves. The survey results indicate that people don't object to methadone maintenance treatment per se, but they object to drug users in general, and heroin users in particular, getting any kind of treatment that might seem to condone their behavior. An unexpected finding was that the older jail staff was much more sympathetic to methadone maintenance treatment, than the younger staff" (McMillan and Lapham, 2005). McMillan's study holds out promise for educating both policymakers and corrections staff who are involved in responding to the health care needs of an inmate population.

Programs for Methadone Treatment of Opioid-Addicted Inmates

There has been considerable experience in providing access to methadone maintenance treatment through an incarcerated population in a major U.S. jail in New York City. The Rikers Island KEEP (Key Extended Entry Program) program has been part of the Rikers Island Health Services System since 1987. This service combines pharmacotherapy and comprehensive therapeutic treatment for heroin addiction.

The KEEP program treats approximately 4,000 inmates with methadone each year, with an average treatment duration of 35 days. Approximately 70 percent of these inmates are men; among women participating in the program, 10 percent are pregnant (Parrino, 2000). To qualify for the KEEP program, an inmate must have been diagnosed as being opioid addicted by medical staff, been charged with either a misdemeanor or low-grade felony, and be serving a misdemeanor sentence. What is most important about this program is that approximately 75 percent of all program participants reported to their assigned outpatient methadone program for continued substance abuse treatment services following their release from jail. This finding, which has been consistent throughout the course of the Rikers Island program, demonstrates clearly that providing treatment to opioid-addicted inmates while they are incarcerated significantly reduces the likelihood of a return to the criminal lifestyle that accompanies illicit heroin use. The KEEP program also demonstrates the value of a tightly coordinated service delivery system between a jail-based program and outpatient methadone treatment programs.

The Rikers Island experience supports both the conclusion of the 1997 NIH Consensus Panel and the National Institute on Drug Abuse's October 1999 *Principles of Drug Addiction Treatment*, which asserts that "research is demonstrating that treatment for drug addicted offenders during and after incarceration can have a significant beneficial effect on future drug use, criminal behavior and social functioning. The case for integrating drug addiction treatment approaches within the criminal justice system is compelling. Combining prison and community-based treatment for drug addiction offenders reduces the risks of both recidivism to drug-related criminal behavior and relapse to drug use" (National Institute on Drug Abuse, 1999).

In spite of growing knowledge that this kind of program should be replicated in jails throughout the U.S. to reduce recidivism at a low cost, the movement to institute such reform has been extremely slow to develop. There is greater likelihood that, in view of their shorter sentences, jail inmates will gain access to continued methadone treatment than will prison inmates. In addition, jails are generally located in communities and counties while prisons tend to be more geographically isolated from the general public. Accordingly, county and municipal jails tend to be more responsive to local political interests.

At the time of this writing, methadone maintenance treatment is offered as a continued form of care in few jails in the U.S. The Orange County Jail in Orlando, Florida, began to provide access to methadone treatment for inmates who were already enrolled in methadone treatment programs at the time of their incarceration following two lawsuits that were very costly to the county. Two of the jail's inmates died from causes medically related to withdrawal symptoms when their methadone treatment was abruptly stopped. Families of the decedents brought the county to court and won significant financial damages. A local methadone treatment program, the Center for Drug-Free Living, now delivers methadone to the Orange County Jail under an agreement between the jail and the treatment program. This arrangement represents an extremely practical solution to a terrible medical crisis for those inmates who are enrolled in a methadone treatment program at time of incarceration and cannot gain access to any effective medical treatment. Several other jail-based methadone treatment programs also provide access to such care, including those in the Philadelphia corrections system, correctional facilities in Rhode Island, and scattered jurisdictions throughout the U.S. New jail-based methadone/buprenorphine–based treatment programs are under consideration in Washington, New Mexico, Maryland, and Vermont.

Emerging Case Law

Legal precedents and case law are limited in this area but are developing. One significant case is that of Keith Griggs, who brought suit against the Vermont Department of Corrections when the department refused to permit access to continued methadone treatment while he was incarcerated. Although the trial judge directed the Vermont Department of Corrections to administer Mr. Griggs's methadone immediately, the department did not do so, instead requesting an emergency stay of the order from the Vermont Supreme Court. The Supreme Court upheld the lower court's ruling. The Vermont Department of Corrections continued to refuse to allow Keith Griggs access to his methadone treatment, and rather than comply with the court order, released Griggs from prison before his sentence had been completed (Boucher, 2003). Boucher's analysis of this and a second similar case from Vermont led her to conclude, "Denying methadone to inmates can no longer pass constitutional muster because it offends the evolving standard of decency that marks the progress of a maturing society, in which scientists have declared opioid dependence a medical disorder treatable with methadone" (Boucher, 2003).

Serving the Needs of Opioid-Addicted Inmates and Society

Several arguments can be made for providing access to methadone/buprenorphine treatment for opioid-addicted inmates in U.S. jails. First, as the NIH Consensus Panel made clear, heroin addiction is a disease for which effective therapy exists. If inmates who suffer from other medical diseases have access to medical care during their incarceration, opioid-addicted inmates should be treated no differently.

Second, methadone/buprenorphine treatment is a low-cost medical intervention. In most outpatient programs, the cost for providing access to this treatment generally amounts to $5,000 per patient per year. This is much lower than the roughly $22,000 per inmate per year cost of incarceration (Boucher, 2003), especially in view of the fact that a large number of methadone patients pay for their own treatment and public costs of correctional systems are steadily rising.

Funding will be needed for jail-based treatment programs, especially as more inmate health care programs are provided under contract with entities in the private sector. The Rikers Island KEEP program has demonstrated that providing access to methadone treatment for inmates is extremely cost effective. The funding needed for jail-based programs, and to support continued access to treatment for opioid-addicted inmates as they leave jail or prison and return to society, could come from federal, state, or county sources.

As McMillan's study shows, attitudes need to be changed in order to increase access to methadone treatment for incarcerated addicts.

But his findings also suggest that attitudes can be changed. And the KEEP program demonstrates that both opioid-addicted individuals and society benefit when inmates have access to treatment for their addiction.

There is no question that society's interests are served by providing opioid-addicted inmates access to methadone and buprenorphine, which are the federally approved medications for treating chronic opioid addiction. In view of the established science in this area of medicine and in view of the cost savings to society, there are no sound arguments against the recommendation to provide access to medications to treat the disease of opioid addiction during the period of an inmate's incarceration.

REFERENCES

Boucher, R. 2003. The case for methadone maintenance treatment in prisons. *Vermont Law Review* 27(2):1–30.

Fiscella, K., Moore, A., Engerman, J., and Meldrum, S. 2004. Jail management of arrestees/inmates enrolled in community methadone maintenance programs. *Journal of Urban Health* 81(4):645–54.

McMillan, G., and Lapham, S. 2005. Staff perspectives on Methadone Maintenance Therapy (MMT) in a large southwestern jail. *Addiction Research and Theory* 13(1):53–63.

National Institutes of Health. 1997. Effective medical treatment of opiate addiction. NIH Consensus Statement Online. November 17–19; 15 (6):1–38 (http://consensus.nih.gov/1997/1998TreatOpiateAddiction1080html.htm).

National Institute on Drug Abuse. 1999. *Principles of Drug Addiction Treatment: A Research-Based Guide*. National Institutes of Health, U.S. Department of Health and Human Services, NIH publication no. 99–4180. Rockville, Md.: National Institute on Drug Abuse.

Parrino, M. 2000. Methadone treatment in jail. *American Jails,* May/June, pp. 9–12.

15

Addiction Art and Science
Two Sides of Humanity

JACK E. HENNINGFIELD, PH.D.,
PATRICIA B. SANTORA, PH.D., AND
WARREN K. BICKEL, PH.D.

Addiction to alcohol, tobacco, illicit drugs, or prescription drugs can happen to anyone. Anyone who has the ability to learn, experience emotions, love, and remember has the biological wiring for addiction. Drugs hijack these basic biological systems and redirect their focus to the drug itself. From a biological perspective, it is an orderly process leading to compulsive and harmful behavior. From a human perspective, it is a disastrous interaction with a powerful substance that alters brain chemistry. A scientific perspective alone can never offer a complete portrayal and understanding of addiction.

In testifying to the U.S. Food and Drug Administration about treatment for tobacco addiction, former Surgeon General C. Everett Koop once said, "It is easy to get the disease but hard to get treatment and our nation must reverse this if we are to move forward" (Koop, 2003, p. 617). He said much the same about HIV/AIDS, adding, "We are fighting a disease and not the people who have it" (see "Introduction," present volume). As a nation we responded much more vigorously to prevent AIDS and to help those with AIDS than we responded to addiction. Why? The challenge was no easier. Yet we seem often to be fighting those with addictions more than we are fighting their disease.

Part of the reason is that the HIV community did a better job of showing the human side of the disease. They enlisted artists and they used art to show us the human side of AIDS. They gave us compassion for those who were afflicted that we could transform into passion to help. Science was called on to provide a path to life, but art gave the reason.

"High on Life: Transcending Addiction" was a major art exhibition in 2002–2003 at the American Visionary Art Museum in Baltimore (American Visionary Art Museum, 2002). As curator Tom Patterson noted, the exhibition presented a "broad spectrum of artists' perspectives on drug use and abuse, altered states of consciousness, addiction recovery, compulsive pleasure-seeking, other forms of compulsive behavior, and related social taboos. The artists come from a wide range of age groups, cultural backgrounds, and social categories, and they address issues of drug use and consciousness in a variety of stimulating, thought-provoking, challenging, and entertaining ways" (Patterson, 2002, p. 19). By showing the human side of addiction, giving those who understand addiction from the inside out opportunity to infuse us with their feelings, their understandings, their needs, and their potential, the exhibition opens the door to the universe of compassion. It is the complementary universe to scientific research. It is as necessary as scientific research because without a passion to understand and to help, the science will go unused.

What Dr. Koop said about tobacco is sadly true for all addictions. Within a few blocks of the museum, drug users can find a "fix," but if they want treatment they must overcome mountainous obstacles. If we are going to help them and reduce the ravages of addiction, we need to stop treating addicted people as though they intend to hurt themselves and others. We need to stop blaming addicted people for their addiction and instead inspire them to seek help. And when they do seek help—as most will—we must ensure that help will be within reach.

Addiction art helps bridge the gap between the science of addiction and the human experience of addiction; it gives insights that no amount of scientific research could. We have included several works of addiction art in this book and hope they will help you see the human side of addiction in all its beauty and tragedy. We hope that you will feel compassion and that you will rise up and say, we need to do more as a city, as a state, as a nation, and as a global community to prevent addiction and help those who are addicted.

ACKNOWLEDGMENT

This chapter was adapted from Henningfield (2002).

REFERENCES

American Visionary Art Museum. 2002. High on Life: Transcending Addiction. *Visions* 8:1–30.

Henningfield, J. E. 2002. Bridge to compassion: a scientist's perspective on addiction and art. *Visions* 8:4–5.

Koop, C. E. 2003. Tobacco addiction: accomplishments and challenges in science, health, and policy. *Nicotine & Tobacco Research* 5:613–19.

Patterson, T. 2002. Curator's notebook. *Visions* 8:18–25.

16

Addiction, Recovery, and Art
My Story

RAYMOND MATERSON

I remember looking around and seeing the clichés of Narcotics Anonymous and Alcoholics Anonymous (*Keep It Simple, Stupid . . . Fake It 'til You Make It*) plastered in large black lettering all around the group room. It was my third (or was it my fourth?) attempt to buy into sobriety. I didn't know, and I didn't care. I didn't care about too much at the time, except, most certainly, whether I could hook up with another druggie to find a good, cheap fix. My eyes wandered around the room, considering candidates.

The people who had found sobriety were apparent to me: the attractive, if somewhat callous-looking, counselor who was chairing the meeting; a bald-headed guy named Joe who was always in need of a shave and invariably referred to himself through a heavy accent as "a stupid Polack with twenty years' sobriety." There were others, too. Some had that look of born-again Christians from a TV evangelist's show. Others sipped coffee and slouched in metal folding chairs, their attire suggesting they were on lunch breaks from minimum-wage jobs, working hard to keep it together but always just a shiver away from slipping off the edge.

Then there were people who were in the same boat I was: we were there because some court had ordered "treatment" or because our families had insisted we get help. But I didn't want help. I was Me. I was somehow special, I told myself, and certainly not like any of these others who surrounded me. Dad had always said we were a different breed. "Don't trust these 'others,'" he would often say. He himself put his faith in no one—like Bogart, who said, "I don't trust anybody, especially dames!" That was Dad.

The clichés pasted on the walls reminded me of my father. He was tragic and bigger than life. He was a drunk. In the throes of his regular binges, he belittled my mother, my sister Barbara, and me to no end. Still, he always provided the necessities of life for us. An educated man, he twisted the words of philosophers and literary giants to fit his diatribes. Thoreau's "Simplicity, simplicity, simplicity" could easily become, "Keep it simple, stupid."

I chuckled to myself. Dad was true to his word yet again: "I'll reach out from the grave to you!" And sure enough, there he was, reaching to me from a two-dimensional crypt on the wall of the unfeeling group room. He was dead, certainly, but he'd never left my side. He was always there no matter what I did or where I found myself. He whispered in my ear continuously: "You're a loser, Raymond"; "You're less than nothing, a gutless double zero."

Over the years it became harder and harder to maintain a confident identity. When I discovered drugs in my early teens, they provided me with something—a borrowed confidence and a false sense of self-esteem. I simultaneously became both a rebel (a trait Dad had extolled) and a cynic. Between these two characteristics, a personality developed that pushed me toward self-destruction.

I don't remember if I ever scored any dope on the day described above. I do know that I didn't learn anything about staying "clean and sober" during my month in treatment. I faked it. When it was over, I got off my ass—in pursuit of the high.

Like torn pages from a stained and brittle family album, the years passed. Eventually, I reached the pinnacle of loserhood: all in the name of staying high and feeling normal, I committed a short string of robberies with a shoplifted toy gun. I was arrested, convicted, and sent to prison.

Prison: it's the home of losers and throwaways. The larger percentage of inmates is there because of substance abuse issues. I recall thinking how ironic it was to watch inmates vying for power and "prestige" in the joint. I laughed to myself at the image of men scrambling and fighting to get on top of each other in that social septic tank, because even when you got on top, you were still reeking of and covered in shit. Prison confirms, minute by agonizing minute, all the worst one has ever thought of oneself. It is the ignoble crowning glory of a life wasted, of having lived with and succumbed to ridicule and abuse. It is not "taking one's medicine."

Let Go and Let God. Sure, I'd seen that one, too. God hadn't answered my prayers when my little, trembling hands dripping with tears were folded in petition asking him to make Daddy stop drinking. He hadn't stood up for me when I'd been falsely accused of vandalizing a school desk in the fourth grade, and he didn't stop the bullies from picking on me for being an A student in junior high. God: an absentee landlord who watched from a long, safe distance as individuals, families, neighborhoods, and entire nations had crumbled and slaughtered themselves and one another since the first sapient creatures crawled out of caves. Still, there had to be someone, some thing, some entity who gave a damn. From my cell in F-Block, none was apparent.

In "The Program" I was told to believe in a Higher Power. I was told to turn my will and my life over to that Higher Power. When a fledgling clean-and-sober wannabe had asked about this Higher Power, a counselor told him it could be Thor the god of thunder or even a doorknob. "Ya need a Higher Power; something bigger than *you* to believe in!" I wasn't quite sure about his references. I was pretty sure God—assuming there was one—looked exactly like the white-bearded Caucasian man sitting in the clouds on a bejeweled throne depicted in my grade school prayer book. Maybe that was okay. I tabled the notion.

It took about a year, 12 or 13 months there in the joint, for me to seriously revisit the concept of God and Higher Power. I'd witnessed fights, stabbings, and humiliations of all variety. I'd managed to stay out of harm's way by keeping to myself. Occasionally, I'd cop a buzz from prison-brewed wine or a few hits off a marijuana bone that a generous fellow inmate offered. The highs were hardly worth the effort.

The occasion of my renewed search for the Divine was the result of listening to a fellow prisoner scream blasphemies and curse God aloud during an absurd argument with another inmate. Somehow, hearing hateful, irreligious spew coming out of the mouth of another human being disturbed me to the core. That night I prayed. I prayed for the doors to be opened. I prayed for a miracle. I believed a miracle could happen.

Somewhat to my surprise, I was not lifted out of my cell by an almighty cosmic force. Nor did the warden show up with the heavenly host and a get-out-of-jail-free card. But over the next week or so, I was mentally inundated with images from my youth. I recalled how much I'd enjoyed school and sports as a child. I remembered with lively reflection how I'd been involved with theater and enjoyed it even as a nine year old. And I remembered my grandmother and her penchant for embroidery.

Grandma had lived with us for a few years when I was small. She had spindly arms and legs as well as a hunchback. When Dad would go into one of his regular tirades, it hardly seemed to bother Grandma as she sat, peacefully embroidering butterflies, flowers, birds, and all variety of designs on tablecloths and pillowcases. I'd never felt terribly close to the old woman, but this was something I'd admired and envied in her. So there in the prison, among murderers, gangsters, thieves, and rapists, I took up the art of embroidery.

Besides colored pencils and pens, the prison offered nothing in the form of arts and craft supplies. My thread was gleaned by unraveling colored socks. My embroidery hoop was improvised from the top of a plastic food-storage container. I borrowed a sewing needle from a friendly prison guard who kept a stash of such items in case an inmate needed to sew a button on a shirt. Slowly I began the process of learning to embroider.

The work consumed virtually all of my waking time. Inmates placed orders for various sports logos, flags, and sentimental images to send to wives, sweethearts, and mothers. A business was born overnight. I was paid for my efforts in "prison money," which typically took the form of cigarettes and bags of coffee, but the pay was secondary to what was taking place inside of me. I was changing. I was beginning to feel good about myself. And with each completed commission, my ability at embroidery grew. I took on challenges. I learned that sewing resembles painting in some respects. I copied the works of master painters and, though I had little experience in drawing and design, I began to create original works.

I listened to classical music on headphones. I reflected on my life, who I was and what I hoped to become. Most important, I began to see that God was not some hairy thunderer, doorknob, or bearded elderly man off in the clouds. I began to see Him as a constant companion, not a distant overseer. God, it seemed, was answering prayers whispered from the corner of the social sewer.

Once I began to see how all things work together for those who believe in miracles and answered prayer, I was open to new growth. A young woman, Melanie, who'd seen works that I'd sent out to my sister, began writing to me. She too had felt betrayed by God as well as family. She too had fallen into the trap of drug abuse. But inside of her were recollections and dreams similar to my own. We began a relationship. First, it was a relationship of encouragement and positive reinforcement. She applauded my art and ideas. I responded in kind by encouraging her creative side and her hopes for her life. Each day was filled with spirit-lifting words; sometimes they came in the form of letters from Melanie, other days they came from the lowliest of my fellow inmates. But they were there. Words that said, "You are worthwhile; you are a good person."

I listened to those words. I soaked them up like a sponge. Like the old socks I was pulling apart and reweaving into miniature artworks, my life was becoming a new and beautiful creation. Good things continued to happen. With Melanie's unwavering support and effort, I received representation in a New York art gallery. My works began to sell and I was sought after by the press. Stories ran on my art and my life in the *New York Times, Sports Illustrated,* and the *Village Voice.* Television news crews came to the prison. It was quite astounding.

With all the positive change in my life, it seemed reasonable to me that the state of Connecticut, where I was imprisoned, should grant me a pardon. An inmate in Connecticut becomes eligible for pardon after serving four years of a sentence. In my case, although I had dozens of letters in support of a pardon, my attempts at securing one were unsuccessful both the first time I applied and the following year. On both occasions I was emotionally crushed. When I received news that my petitions had been denied, I felt like giving up. If drugs had been readily available to me, I believe I would have used. Then it occurred to me: they say in the AA program that if you spent 10, 15, or 20 years becoming an out-of-control drunk, it's going to take the same amount of time to undo the damage and craziness. It could only have been that God, my Higher Power, knew better for me.

Despite the letdown, which Melanie and I worked through via letters, phone calls, and visits, we continued to move forward. There were art shows to plan for and, most notably, a wedding. In the spring of 1993, Melanie and I exchanged vows. We also began talking about "what went right" in my recovery from addiction. We talked about the spiritual roots of addiction and self-destructive behavior. A somewhat simple cause was hypothesized: people are born with an innate drive to create, build, and explore their personal abilities. If this is not nurtured and encouraged, the tendency is to turn toward the opposite: personal stagnation and destructiveness. The destructiveness can take the form of self-destructive behaviors, such as drug addiction, or can be turned outward at others.

Although the theory may seem far too anecdotal for some, I have come to believe that restoring a person's self-esteem is imperative in helping him or her overcome addiction. I also believe that the spiritual awakening or reawakening of the individual is a necessary and essential aspect of recovery. I don't recommend worshiping Thor or doorknobs, but an exploration of the spiritual is an undeniable part of personal growth and continued sobriety. I know this because I have seen it work in my own life.

Finally, treatment takes time. Great ideas, epiphanies, and "light bulb" moments may happen in the head in a twinkling. But, to quote Humphrey Bogart again, "When your head says one thing and your whole life says something else, your head loses." Twenty-eight-day recovery programs are revolving doors. For many addicts, treatment needs to include long-term residential care. If the government can build prisons and keep more than 2 million people behind bars, the government can't afford not to subsidize long-term treatment facilities for the poor, the homeless, and those most at risk for ending up in the criminal justice system. Treatment on demand for addicts must be the rule, not the dream.

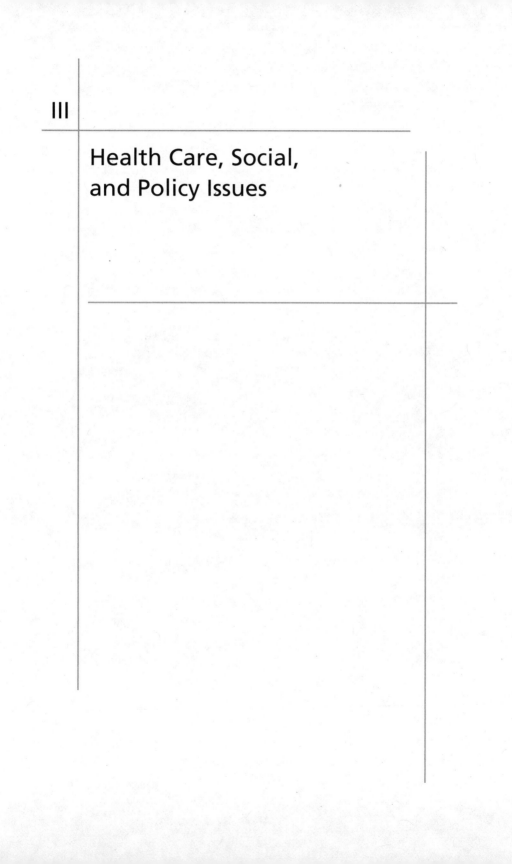

III

Health Care, Social, and Policy Issues

17

Advancing the Science Base for the Treatment of Addiction

ALAN I. LESHNER, PH.D.

Advances in science over the past 30 years have revolutionized our fundamental understanding of drug abuse and addiction and what to do about them. Science has taught that, whatever their social causes and concomitants, drug abuse and addiction are fundamentally health issues, certainly when examined at the level of individual drug users and addicts. For that reason, any national strategies for dealing with them must include substantial focus on prevention and treatment. In fact, many have argued that the current balance in both policy and funding between criminal justice and health approaches is inappropriate and that it should be readjusted to favor more emphasis on treatment, prevention, and research. Unfortunately, ideology and intuition continue to drive much of drug addiction policy and practice, and therefore there is a substantial gap between what the science suggests and most national and local strategies for dealing with these issues.

What the Science Says

We now know that prolonged drug use changes brain structure and function in ways that result in compulsive, typically uncontrollable drug craving, seeking, and use, the condition we call addiction. Addiction is, thus, at its core a brain disease—a disease that comes about because of a behavior (drug use), is expressed in behavioral ways (compulsive drug use), and is dependent on the social context in which it occurs. The reason that addicts cannot simply will themselves to stop using drugs is that they are in an altered brain state (Leshner, 2001; Volkow and Li, 2004).

We have learned that the old distinctions between "physical" (often called "physiological") and "psychological" addiction are no longer appropriate. First, the compulsion to use drugs emerges in large part from biological changes. What used to be called "psychological addiction" is just as physiological in nature as what we now call "physical dependence," the condition characterized by the dramatic bodily changes that accompany withdrawal from drugs such as heroin and alcohol. Second, stopping use of many of the most addicting substances (crack cocaine, methamphetamine) does not result in florid physical withdrawal symptoms. The fact that a substance does or does not cause physical dependence is irrelevant to how powerfully addictive it is.

Advances in science, in this case coupled with much clinical experience, have also provided an array of quite effective drug addiction treatments. These addiction treatments have passed scientific tests of effectiveness that are as rigorous as those demonstrating effectiveness for treatments for other chronic, relapsing disorders, like hypertension, diabetes, and asthma (McLellan et al., 2000). The best treatment strategies are directed at the whole person, because addiction hijacks all aspects of one's life, including virtually all of the individual's social interactions. Whole-person treatments include biological, behavioral, and social components, typically including medication when available, individual psychotherapy, group therapy, family therapy, vocational rehabilitation, and so on (National Institute on Drug Abuse, 1999).

Superb Science

Drug addiction research now ranks among the best and most productive in modern science. For example, studies of the molecular and cellular mechanisms of drug action have helped set the high standards and have stimulated much research about more general aspects of signal transduction and gene expression. Studies of the mechanisms of drug reward and reinforcement have taught a great amount about motivational processes more generally.

Addiction studies have been among the most productive of all in the brain-imaging field, and they have taught much about more general aspects of brain-mind interactions. As one example, much further research on impulse control deficits in other conditions has been stimulated directly by clinical neurobiological studies of addiction. Technology developments to facilitate addiction imaging studies—such as new positron-emission technology (or PET) scan ligands or functional magnetic resonance imaging (or fMRI) approaches—have been extremely useful for understanding other aspects of human brain structure and function.

This great progress in drug abuse research has been accelerated by the same kinds of technology developments that have been dramatically advancing the rest of biomedical science. These include new approaches to information and computational sciences, new molecular genetic techniques, and brain imaging (Volkow et al., 2003). The ability to observe directly what is going on in the human brain during mental events has elucidated much about the neurobiological bases of both the compulsion itself and about other addiction-related phenomena, like the nature of the drug experience and the brain expression of drug craving during abstinence. Moreover, it is clear that progress in addiction research is as dependent on progress in the mathematical, physical, and chemical sciences as are other areas of the life sciences. The cutting edge of virtually all fields is multidisciplinary in nature, and one could argue that traditional disciplines are by now only administrative conveniences (Leshner, 2004).

The Gaps among Science, Practice, and Public Policy

In light of this superb base of scientific understanding, why have both public perceptions and national policies lagged so far behind the science? The answers likely lie in public and policymaker attitudes, not in conflicting facts. One overarching attitudinal issue is the tremendous stigma that surrounds all aspects of drug abuse and addiction. Historically, people have disdained addicts because they thought addicts "did it to themselves" and could just quit if they really wanted to. Moreover, addiction does cause a great amount of familial and broader social disruption. Many members of the public also have believed that the people who work with addicts are amateurs, just former addicts themselves, and they have thought that people who study addicts cannot work on "real problems." None of that is true, of course, and advances in science have helped destigmatize addiction and addiction workers, but we still have a long way to go in changing public attitudes toward both our patients and our professionals.

A second, related counterweight to science-based approaches is ideology—both within and outside the drug addiction field. Within the field, many addiction workers are loath to give up long-held but nonscientific views of both the origins of and ways to treat addiction. Many programs retain prevention or treatment components that began as someone's bright idea, seemed to work pretty well, and by now have acquired an almost superstitious aura of validity. Because those components have never been subjected to scientific tests to establish or disprove their efficacy, the programs see no clear reason to discard them, even though there also is no clear reason to keep them. Moreover, many treatment organizations do not have sufficient numbers of trained personnel to scour the scientific literature on a regular basis, and thus they are not familiar with the latest science of drug addiction and its treatment.

Ideology and intuition underpin most views of drug abuse and addiction held by the general public. Seventy million adult Americans have used an illegal drug at some point in their lives. Many think that they are experts simply as a result of their personal experiences, similar to how many people feel about education—they went to school themselves, so they feel free to tell their children's teachers how to teach. For example, a large number of people have experimented with drugs a few times and many of them were easily able to stop using. Why can't addicts do the same? They and their friends smoked quite a lot of marijuana, by their standards, and did not become addicted; how can we say marijuana can be addicting? In relation to this, as mentioned above, the fact that addiction begins with the voluntary behavior of drug use makes it difficult for many in the general public to believe that addicts really cannot just stop their drug use without treatment; they simply must not be sufficiently motivated.

The social and criminal justice concomitants of drug use and addiction—such as family disruption, street crime, and the like—also make many people feel that addicts need to be punished, not offered treatment for their drug use. It does not matter that the data show that simply incarcerating addicts without drug treatment is virtually a guarantee of their returning to both drug use and crime, whereas treating addicts while they are under criminal justice control significantly reduces both forms of recidivism (Cornish et al., 1997; Butzin et al.,

2002). What seems to matter most is that the offender is punished for his or her criminal behavior. To many people, treating addicted offenders is equal to coddling them.

How can we move forward? Much of the responsibility lies with the scientific community, which must do a far better job of publicizing its work. Scientists must explain their findings in easily understood terms that clarify the importance and potential impact of their research. Drug abuse prevention and treatment practitioners should reach out more to the people in their local communities. In the process, however, they need to give up some of the off-putting jargon that has so long characterized our field and talk about what science has taught about their patients, the nature of their illness, and about the science base for prevention and treatment. Policymakers and political leaders must have the courage to rethink their own overarching biases about the issues and to develop new strategic approaches that follow the science. With focused collective effort and with sufficient will, science can replace ideology as the foundation for how we approach drug abuse and addiction and become far more effective in dealing with them.

REFERENCES

Butzin, C. A., Martin, S. S., and Inciardi, J. A. 2002. Evaluating component effects of a prison-based treatment continuum. *Journal of Substance Abuse Treatment* 22:66–69.

Cornish, J. W., Metzger, D., Woody, G. E., Wilson, D., McLellan, A. T., Vandergrift, B., and O'Brien, C. P. 1997. Naltrexone pharmacotherapy for opioid dependent federal probationers. *Journal of Substance Abuse Treatment* 14:529–34.

Leshner, A. I. 2001. Addiction is a brain disease. *Issues in Science and Technology* 17:75–80.

Leshner, A. I. 2004. Science at the leading edge. *Science* 303:729.

McLellan, A. T., Lewis, D. C., O'Brien, C. P., and Kleber, H. D. 2000. Drug dependence, a chronic medical illness. *JAMA* 284:1689–95.

National Institute on Drug Abuse. 1999. *Principles of Drug Addiction Treatment: A Research-Based Guide.* Bethesda, Md.: National Institute on Drug Abuse.

Volkow, N. D., and Li, T.-K. 2004. Drug addiction: the neurobiology of behaviour gone awry. *Nature Reviews, Neuroscience* 5:963–70.

Volkow, N. D., Fowler, J. S., and Wang, G.-J. 2003. The addicted human brain: insights from imaging studies. *Journal of Clinical Investigation* 111:1444–51.

18

"Going Upstream"
Thoughts for Substance Abuse Professionals

LAWRENCE WALLACK, DR.P.H.

Alcohol, tobacco, and other drugs continue to take a terrible toll on American society. Whether the metric is dollars, lost opportunities, dreams shattered, or lives lost, the tragedy is all the greater because so much of it is preventable. The field of substance abuse prevention and treatment has the benefit of bright, determined, and tireless people at all levels of science, education, advocacy, policy, and service provision. Because our goal is so important, our challenge so great, and our resources so limited, however, it is not surprising that a slow rate of progress is often mistaken for a lack of progress. We would do well to heed the advice of Marty Mann, one of the first women to join Alcoholics Anonymous: "We need to appreciate how far we have come, and not just focus on how far we still have to go."

The problems posed by substance abuse are deeply woven into our social fabric. The causes and solutions of substance abuse cut across all levels, from deep within the individual to the broad and abstract values and norms that connect us as a society. Nonetheless, advances in policy, science, and sophisticated organizing by the activist community have saved lives and allowed dreams to be realized.

How can we ensure continued progress? Let's consider four points: developing an upstream vision, identifying some basic principles to guide us, thinking about the nature of social justice, and tapping a deeper spiritual connection.

Developing an Upstream Vision

What is an upstream vision? Think of it this way: A group of people is standing alongside a river. Suddenly there is a cry for help from a drowning person in the water. One of the bystanders jumps into the water and drags the person to shore, and then another starts to give mouth-to-mouth resuscitation. Someone else is berating the rescued individual for not being a better swimmer and another is offering discount coupons for swimming lessons. Suddenly there is another cry for help and the rescue is repeated. This goes on with more and more people needing to be rescued. Finally, someone realizes the futility of constantly saving drowning swimmers one by one and turns to her colleague and says, "We are so busy pulling people out of the water that we aren't able to go upstream and find out why they are falling in the river." So they leave behind those who are blaming others for not being good swimmers and strike out up the river to look at why so many are falling in the river. They have embarked on the search for root causes.

Downstream work is important and can help many people. But remember, unless we reduce the number of people falling into the river upstream we will never solve the problem of people needing to be rescued downstream. Our workload will only increase. It will get worse, not better, because we cannot pull people out of the river faster than they are falling or being pushed in.

Upstream is the state of mind needed to make a difference, but it is not easy, because we are a downstream society. We seem more willing to intervene when problems are already firmly established, suffering already in place, and the cost is great than to invest in prevention. Certainly, we have been more willing to build costly prisons than invest in schools. We invest more in punishment than in education; we have been more interested in funding incarceration than in finding prevention programs that work.

Identifying Guiding Principles

What are some important principles or values that might help us to find our way upstream?

We need to understand that we are all in this together. We are part of an interconnected system in which the wellbeing of the individual is linked to the wellbeing of the community. Similarly, individual behavior cannot be fully understood and addressed absent the context of the larger society in which it takes place. It is not only our individual behavior but the behavior of our major social institutions that matter.

We need to ask more challenging questions. In *Gravity's Rainbow,* Thomas Pynchon wrote, "If they can get you asking the wrong questions, the answers don't matter." Think about that. We need to ask the right questions, the hard questions about how the burdens of prevention should be shared, how accountability for substance abuse should be determined.

We share responsibility collectively for problems and their solutions, and we have a strong obligation to serve the collective good. This sense of obligation to the collective good is the heart of our communities and the greatness of our democracy.

Scientific inquiry must be the basis for an informed, rational public debate about the problems we face. Facts must matter, and research has to count.

Basic benefits such as affordable housing, health care, education, and living-wage jobs should be assured, so families can take advantage of opportunities for upward mobility.

Government involvement is necessary to remedy the limits and abuses of the market, whether it takes the form of limiting tobacco advertising aimed at youth, providing treatment to those in need, or limiting availability of alcohol in high-risk settings. The issue is better government, not bigger or smaller government.

Thinking about Social Justice

How can we get our heads around such a concept as vast as social justice?

In his classic work *A Theory of Justice,* John Rawls writes about justice as fairness. He argues that we should select the principles of justice that will guide our actions as objectively as we can. To do that, we must envision ourselves in an "original position" in which there are no preexisting rules and think about what would be fair from behind a "veil of ignorance" where we do not know our own status. This is an interesting thought experiment.

Imagine that you do not know whether you would be born rich or poor; man or woman; in Japan, with the world's longest life expectancy, or Sierra Leone, where life expectancy is among the shortest in the world, at only 26 years; whether you have all your physical and mental capabilities or few or none; whether you were born into the best neighborhood or the worst housing project; whether you were a chain smoker, a heroin addict, or an alcoholic. Now imagine, given this veil of ignorance, how you would select the guiding principles for society that you think are fair, how you would design policies about the economy, jobs, globalization, education, health, housing, and social programs. What would you want the rules of society to be if you did not know where and how you would begin? How level would you want the playing field to be?

Tapping a Deeper Spiritual Connection

What about the spiritual dimension? This concerns the interconnection of all things at a deep level. And today, perhaps more than ever before, there are reminders everywhere. On the physical level there is the slowly dawning realization that we all share the air we breathe, the water we drink, the atmosphere above us, the oceans that surround us. Microbes travel across the ocean in a few hours, hitching a ride with an unsuspecting airline passenger and suddenly we are experiencing the same symptoms as another human many miles away. The omnipresent Internet allows us to connect in a moment with someone on the other side of the planet. For many of us these reminders that we are interdependent come to us many times each day. The choices we make in this country will continue to affect the realities of life in other parts of the world. And always beneath the aspirations for a good life, however that may be defined around the world, lie those big questions. We search for meaning and seek to understand how our individual lives fit into some larger picture. We seek opportunities to love and to be loved.

It's also about compassion. Compassion is something we need to have for ourselves as well as for others. The ability to learn and move on when things do not turn out as we had planned them. The trust that it is all part of something bigger.

Compassion toward others is about how wide and inclusive we make the circle of compassion—is it expansive or narrow, does it apply to the few or to many, to those who may hold values different from our own as well as those who share our values? When you are drawing your circle of compassion, consider the words of Chief Seattle, the great Sioux warrior: "This we know: the earth does not belong to man, man belongs to the earth. All things are connected like the blood that unites us all. Man did not weave the web of life; he is merely a strand in it. Whatever he does to the web, he does to himself."

The field of substance abuse prevention and treatment is on the right track, but we need to be sure we are traveling in the right direction—that direction is upstream. If you cannot do it in your actions, you must do it in your thinking. We need to link what is happening in our clinics, schools, community organizations, and chambers of public policy to our greater purpose as a national community. Ultimately, upstream is the direction of justice, fairness, equal opportunity, and compassion.

A society that effectively structures itself around an upstream ethic and reflects this in public policy will be a society that better understands the meaning of public health and responds more appropriately to its challenges. It will certainly be a society that more effectively and more humanely addresses the tragedy of substance abuse in the twenty-first century.

ACKNOWLEDGMENT

The author is indebted to his wife, Linda Nettekoven, for her inspiration in writing this chapter.

19

In Praise of Stigma

SALLY SATEL, M.D.

A few years ago, a journalist asked me whether I was concerned about the stigma associated with addiction. I replied that I could imagine few behaviors more deserving of stigmatization. The National Association of Alcohol and Drug Abuse Counselors greeted my comment with a press release stating, "Dr. Satel's nonsensical statement that divorces brain functioning from human behavior further erodes her credibility as an addiction expert."[1] Some months later, I repeated my prostigma comment at a debate at the annual meeting of the College on Problems of Drug Dependence and elicited a collective gasp from the audience.

Clearly, I committed heresy.

Fighting stigma is all the rage nowadays. But the stigma abolitionists rarely say what exactly it is they wish to strip of shame: addictive behavior, seeking help, or addiction treatment itself? I vigorously applaud help-seeking; encourage attendance at a twelve-step group; and believe treatment should be accessible, respectful, and competent. But we don't have to neutralize the moral valence of addiction-fueled behavior to destigmatize the treatment process. We approve of bad parents and abusive spouses when they try to improve themselves through therapy without ever condoning their abusiveness. Indeed, I think it is bad policy to try to cleanse the addict's image. Why try to destigmatize irresponsibility that leads to ruptured families, ruined careers, and crime? Besides, it is unlikely the public would go along; just look at the justifiably scornful attitudes toward drunk drivers.

Let us consider some of the alleged benefits of eliminating stigma, as set forth by the National Institute on Drug Abuse.[2]

Eliminating stigma will get more addicts into treatment. Consider the employee with a drug problem who wants time off to enter treatment. He is reluctant to ask his boss, lest he feel embarrassed or suffer some kind of reprisal. In the end, the worker does not ask for leave, he does not get treatment, and his drug problem worsens. If he had a bad hip, instead of drug problem, the employee would not have hesitated to ask for leave to undergo surgery.

Yet for every employee who is ashamed to tell his boss or fears some kind of reprisal, another may decide to stop on his own or get help precisely because he wants to avoid the embarrassment of failing at the job or of revealing the problem to his boss. Shame, or the prospect of experiencing it, can be an effective deterrent. "Eliminating stigma" may backfire by making more addicts comfortable continuing drug use and avoiding treatment.

Eliminating stigma will improve the availability of treatment. Another rationale for promoting the idea that addiction is simply a medical condition—comparable to, say, hypertension or asthma—is to increase public and political will to fund drug treatment. Greater availability of treatment is a worthy goal, indeed, though I am skeptical that antistigma campaigns of the "have-you-hugged-an-addict-today?" variety will help. Surely, patients must not be discharged from treatment prematurely, but whether a revolving door should be kept open for those who relapse repeatedly—a behavior almost always under one's control—is highly debatable. (The same is true of non-compliant patients with diabetes, for example. Perhaps, they too, should come under more scrutiny for poor self-care.) Softening the moral dimension of addiction is not why we divert petty drug criminals to treatment instead of jail. The reason drug courts have exploded since the early 1990s is because their architects were hard-headed enough to predict that supervised treatment is more effective and less expensive than incarceration—not because treatment is kinder and gentler than jail—and subsequent outcome analyses vindicated their hypothesis.

Eliminating stigma will speed the development of medications. Unlikely. Potential for commercialization will eventually trump bad press—cynical perhaps, but true. After all, consider the innovation in HIV/AIDS drugs. Although male-on-male sex and intravenous drug use—the main vehicles for transmission of HIV—have negative moral connotations, that has not stopped companies from undertaking robust research and development programs on antiviral medications. If there are few antiaddiction medications in the pipeline, it is because few show clinical promise. If a blockbuster drug for addiction comes along, the me-toos will soon come roaring down the pipeline.

Eliminating stigma will help addicts' "self-esteem." Is this necessarily a good thing? In my clinic, many patients say they came for help only because they "couldn't stand" themselves any longer. Why insulate individuals from the adverse consequences of their behavior when those consequences (a) motivate them to seek help and (b) serve as a lesson to others about socially acceptable conduct?[3] And what would substance prevention counselors do if they couldn't warn youth about the consequences of alcohol and drug abuse? Consequences are meant to strike teens as aversive precisely because they signify a moral lapse or portend humiliation.

In sum, the goals of destigmatization listed above are noble (except, perhaps, the desire to protect addicts' "self-esteem," which is just naive). But no matter how many times we hear that "addiction is a brain disease" or are shown illuminated positron emission tomography scans of addicts' craving brains, it will not change the fact that the *behavior* of addicted people is what the public condemns. Indeed, as one of my colleagues put it, you can examine brains all day, but you would never call anyone an addict unless he acted like one.

But can he control how he acts? Yes. The phrase "brain disease" implies otherwise, yet there is much that is indeed voluntary in addiction.

Contingency management experiments in the lab and in the clinic show that rewards and sanctions typically exert a significant effect on drug use. This is the very essence of voluntariness: the course of a behavior can be intentionally altered in response to consequences. No amount of reinforcement or punishment can alter the course of a truly autonomous biological condition. Imagine bribing a cancer patient—one who adhered faithfully to the treatment regimen prescribed by her physician—to keep her tumor from metastasizing or threatening her with jail if her tumor spread.

In the midst of intense craving, granted, it is very hard to govern oneself. Addicts, however, do not spend all of their time in such a state. In the days between binges, for example, cocaine addicts make many deliberate choices, and one of those choices could be the choice to stop using the drug. Heroin-dependent individuals, by comparison, use the drug several times a day but can often function quite well as long as they have stable access to some form of opiate drug to prevent withdrawal symptoms. What's more, addicts have episodes of clean time that last for weeks, months, or years. During these periods, it is their responsibility to reduce vulnerability to drug craving and relapse.

Motivation and self-control are acts of the brain as well. Psychologist Gene Heyman, at McLean Hospital, in Massachusetts, makes a subtle but powerful point when he reminds us that voluntary behavior is also mediated by the brain (Heyman, 2003). If we somehow removed stigma we would effectively decrease opportunities to treat the brain insofar as decisions to change depend on a cognitive calculus that often includes the desire to minimize shame. The question is not whether the brain is involved in addiction or whether compulsive drug use changes brains, but whether addicts' behavior can be influenced by its consequences (i.e., is voluntary). The answer is that it can.

When antistigma champions bemoan the fact that "substance abuse is seen as a personal failing or lack of willpower," they don't seem to realize that recovery itself depends on willpower—and thank goodness it does.[4] Acknowledging as much does not "blame the victim," but rather it endorses an optimistic truth that people have the capacity to transform themselves. Alcoholics Anonymous leverages this logic when it says one is not responsible for being an alcoholic (that is, for inheriting or developing a disorder of control) but one is responsible for not drinking.

In the end, the destigmatization campaign—whose practical aims are to encourage people with substance problems to get care and to ensure that treatment is available to them—has its heart in the right place. But its goals will come about, I believe, only when the effectiveness of treatment itself improves. This will boost the public's perception of its value and increase demand, and for this to happen we need good quality care with better treatment outcomes. Former addicts themselves—the treatment beneficiaries—must become visible symbols of hard work and responsibility. In a sense, they must destigmatize themselves; it is not something a slogan can achieve. All of this is difficult.

Promulgating antistigma rhetoric is easy, not to mention a feel-good waste of time. Keith Humphries, a psychologist at Stanford University, offers a good analogy in the form of Americans' initial attitudes toward immigrant groups, like the Irish, Italian, Jews and Koreans. Contempt for them did abate after time—not because of ads and posters but because they succeed in America, and success destigmatizes.

Finally, even if we could somehow untaint addiction, what would be the price? Stigmatization is a normal part of human interaction, has a civilizing effect on social life, and is often the basis of the antidrug messages we give to children. Censure and disapproval can help define deviancy upward (to play on Daniel Patrick Moynihan's famous phrase), causing drug users to hit their moral bottom sooner so that, finally, they stop using or go into treatment. There is nothing unethical—and everything natural and socially adaptive—about condemning the reckless and harmful behaviors that addicts commit. This need not negate our sympathy for them or our duty to provide care.

NOTES

1. Letter dated May 1, 2003, www.weird-harolds.com/print.php?sid=44.

2. www.drugabuse.gov/about/welcome/aboutdrugabuse/stigma/

3. I do not consider harm reduction techniques (e.g., needle exchange, methadone) to be at odds with this notion. By the time individuals require/want these services, they are already exhibiting behaviors that are socially distasteful.

4. National Governors Association, www.nga.org/center/divisions/1,1188,C_ISSUE_BRIEF/vD_4407,00.html.

REFERENCE

Heyman, G. M. 2003. Consumption dependent changes in reward value: A framework for understanding addiction. In N. Heather and R. Vuchinich, eds., *Choice, Behavioral Economics, and Addiction.* New York: Elsevier.

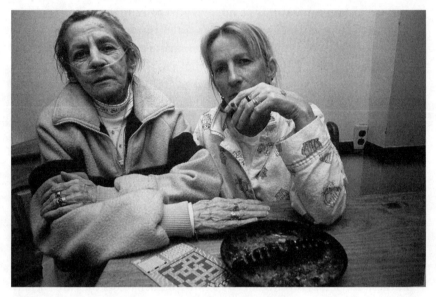

"Kayla's Ma and Grandma," by Brenda Ann Kenneally

20

Addiction as Disease
Policy, Epidemiology, and Treatment Consequences of a Bad Idea

STANTON PEELE, PH.D., J.D.

The effect of conceptualizing addiction as a disease on policy and treatment has been predictably disastrous. The disease conception that addiction can only become progressively worse and never self-ameliorate is decisively wrong. Accepting this misconception leads to the belief that addictions can be remedied only through treatment when, in fact, natural recovery is typical. Moreover, treatment predicated on the notion of addiction as a disease treats those who are addicted as though they were unable to affect their own outcomes (represented by the twelve-step idea of powerlessness). The most effective treatments, by contrast, convey greater power and self-control (i.e., self-efficacy) to addicts and understand that environmental conditions and skills at coping with them are crucial to remission. In the policy realm, the view that addiction inevitably requires treatment leads to support for coercion into treatment, usually twelve-step treatment. At the broader cultural level, the highest incidence of addiction occurs where there is widespread cultural belief in the disease model of addiction.

Policy amid the Consensus That Addiction Is a Disease

The idea that addiction is a disease has become almost received wisdom among conservatives and liberals alike. For example, people on both sides of the drug policy debate—those who favor continued repressive measures toward drug use and those who feel drug laws should be relaxed—agree in this view. Those who favor maintaining the status quo believe that any drug use causes irreversible compulsive drug use, whereas those who favor changing drugs' legal status want to offer compulsive drug users treatment in place of criminal sanctions. At the same time, accepting addiction as a disease means ignoring important views held by those on both ends of the political spectrum. Conservatives who advocate the disease model neglect the ideas of responsibility and self-determination that are part of the conservative model of behavior, and liberals accept that people cannot control their drug use even though this view infantilizes drug users and places them under institutional and state control, contrary to the essential liberal view that humans can and should control their destinies.

These contradictions present fundamental dilemmas for conservatives and liberals. If conservatives accept that drug use can be an uncontrollable disease, they open up the possibility of addiction as a criminal defense—"Once I began using drugs, I could not choose to stop or control my behavior while addicted or intoxicated." Liberals meanwhile, including drug policy reformers, sacrifice the idea that many people are able to control their drug use or that, even when addicted, people are human beings who should be allowed to make choices for themselves. They make this sacrifice to allow those caught using drugs—regardless of whether they are addicted—the option of being treated rather than incarcerated. In this framework, treatment is coercively foisted on people because it is perceived to be a humane alternative to other criminal penalties. The idea that people cannot help themselves out of addiction, however, undermines the very cultural beliefs that are associated with lower rates of addiction.

The Epidemiology of Addictive Drug Use

There are two worlds of addiction: the one glimpsed through clinical dealings with addicts and the one viewed through broad population, epidemiologic studies (Room, 1980). At times, these two worlds are almost unrecognizably different. In the clinical world, patients require constant attention and direction, hardly ever make progress, at least without tremendous therapeutic support and input, and must abstain. In the epidemiologic survey world, treatment is unusual yet addicts usually improve, often gradually, over years, though they are not fixated on abstinence.

Table 20.1. NESARC Past-Year Drinking among Alcoholics

Past-Year Status	Treated ($n=1,205$)	Untreated ($n=3,217$)
Dependent	28	24
Abstinent	35	12
Partial remission	20	30
Remission, risk drinking	6	14
Remission, drinking without risk	10	20

Source: Dawson et al. (2005).

There are many clinics but few massive epidemiologic studies, so we only periodically get the broad view the latter reveal. The results of such studies are stunning, even to professionals, yet they are generally quickly forgotten. In 2005 the National Institute on Alcohol Abuse and Alcoholism (NIAAA) published the results of its 2001–2002 National Epidemiologic Survey on Alcohol and Related Conditions (NESARC), a comprehensive survey focused on Americans' current and lifetime alcohol and drug use (Dawson et al., 2005). NESARC replicated a similar study, the National Longitudinal Alcohol Epidemiologic Survey, conducted a decade earlier that yielded comparable results (cf. Dawson, 1996). NESARC conducted 43,093 in-person interviews with a national sample of adults (18 or older), among whom, at some point prior to the past year, 4,422 were classifiable as alcohol dependent according to DSM-IV. (Because it remains an evocative and popular term, we will refer to this group as "alcoholics.") The NESARC results are presented in Table 20.1.

The first startling finding from NESARC is that only about a quarter of those ever identified as having been alcohol dependent according to DSM-IV criteria were ever treated (including attending Alcoholics Anonymous [AA]). In addition, a higher percentage of treated than untreated alcoholics currently continue to be alcoholic! Twenty-eight percent of those who have received treatment remain dependent, as opposed to 24 percent of those who were never treated. This could partly be accounted for in that treated subjects tend to be more severely alcohol dependent than untreated alcoholics (though the populations overlap). Nonetheless, it is surely embarrassing to an American agency responsible for ameliorating alcoholism that people treated for their alcoholism are no more likely to overcome their alcohol dependence than alcoholics who are not treated.

Those who are treated are substantially more likely to be abstinent (by a three-to-one ratio). The nonabstinence categories in NESARC require some explanation. "Partial remission" refers to alcoholics who had at least one drinking problem over the prior 12 months but who do not qualify for a DSM-IV diagnosis of alcohol dependence. There are, furthermore, two remission-with-drinking categories. The NESARC report identifies one group as "risk drinkers in remission." They have displayed no drinking problems over the prior year, yet they have continued to drink regularly (averaging more than 14 drinks per week for men; 7 drinks per week for women), or they had a single day (or more) in the past year in which they had 5 or more drinks, for men; 4 or more, for women.

Considering a former alcoholic who has had four drinks once in the past year—a year with no alcohol-related work, health, family, or psychological problems—to be a risk drinker might be considered importing a clinical idea into the epidemiological realm. That is, if someone who has been alcohol dependent is now able to get through an entire year with no drinking problems, but periodically (even if extremely rarely) consumes a number of drinks, the person might seem extremely well inured against a return to alcoholism. A clinician, on the other hand, sees the person dancing on the precipice of a fall into an uncontrollable resumption of alcoholism. In fact, it seems likely that opposition from those with a clinical perspective within and outside the NIAAA prompted NESARC investigators to create this risk category (which was not a part of the analysis of remission in NLAES; see Dawson, 1996).

Discarding this add-on to DSM-IV criteria, the NESARC results become even more startling and controversial. Categorizing NESARC respondents purely in terms of their DSM-IV remission categories (Table 20.2) makes clear that untreated alcoholics are more than twice as likely to be in remission while continuing to drink as are treated alcoholics. In fact, the *typical* form remission takes for the large majority of Americans who do not seek treatment for their alcoholism is controlled drinking (by a margin of almost three to one versus abstinence). At the same time, many might be surprised to see that even 16 percent of treated alcoholics achieve nonabstinent remission, or almost half as many as abstain.

Table 20.2. NESARC Past-Year Remission among Alcoholics

Past-Year Status	Treated ($n = 1,205$)	Untreated ($n = 3,217$)
Dependent	28	24
Abstinent	35	12
Partial remission	20	30
Drinking remission	16	34

Source: Dawson et al. (2005).

Table 20.3. NESARC Past-Year Improvement among Alcoholics

Past-Year Status	Treated ($n = 1,205$)	Untreated ($n = 3,217$)
Dependent	28	24
Abstinent	35	12
Drinking without dependence	36	64

Source: Dawson et al. (2005).

Indeed, the NESARC data in Table 20.3—subjects who remain dependent, who cease drinking altogether, or who improve beyond dependence while continuing to drink—represent results that the NIAAA (along with virtually all American clinical authorities) would disavow. Even among those who receive treatment, as many alcoholics improve by drinking with fewer problems as achieve abstinence. Among alcoholics who do not seek treatment, almost two-thirds make such progress. Considering both the treated and untreated populations, the *typical* outcome of alcoholism in the United States is to improve while continuing to drink. The good news is that the majority of alcoholic Americans ignore the disease theory's prescription of abstinence, and they gain benefits from doing so. *Alcoholics who have been in treatment, however, are significantly impaired in their ability to moderate their drinking, whether because of their drinking problems or attitudes prior to being in treatment or as a result of treatment.* Rudy (1986) describes the process of AA members learning, and imitating, the symptoms of full-blown alcoholism that many did not originally display.

Through the Substance Abuse and Mental Health Services Administration (SAMHSA), the United States also conducts a periodic com-

Table 20.4. Lifetime, Past-Month Use of "Addictive" Drugs, United States, 2002

	Percentage of Americans Using (figures rounded)		
	Lifetime	Previous Month	Previous Month/ Lifetime
Cocaine	15	1	7
Crack	3	0.3	9
Heroin	2	0.1	6

Source: Data from SAMHSA (2003, Table 1.1B).

prehensive examination of Americans' drug use, the National Survey on Drug Use and Health. According to this survey, only a small percentage (fewer than 10 percent) of Americans who have ever consumed heroin, crack, or cocaine continue to take these drugs, even as infrequently as once a month (Table 20.4). Presumably, only a small percentage of these "current users" use the drugs addictively. These broad population data defy the commonplace classification of notoriously "addictive" drugs as being distinctively addictive relative to other activities people engage in or substances they consume.

Other epidemiological research, for example with cocaine, indicates that in untreated populations those whose cocaine use leads to physical (e.g., nasal bleeding), psychological (paranoia), and behavioral (e.g., sleep disruption) problems *typically* respond by quitting or cutting back (Erickson et al., 1987; Peele and DeGrandpre, 1998). None of these data discount that some individuals undergo extended periods of excessive, even compulsive use, but this is not true for the large majority of users, even after they encounter substantial problems.

How Belief Systems Influence Levels of Addiction

Attitudes about whether addiction (and alcoholism) is a disease and what that means do not occur in a vacuum; they reflect larger cultural attitudes and belief systems that actually impact whether people control intoxicant-related behavior (Peele, 1985). Cultures in which a drug experience is seen as being overwhelming and insurmountable in fact make addiction to that experience more likely (Peele, 1985). For some time, substantial cultural differences in drinking patterns have been reported in observational studies, often anthropological (cf.

Heath, 2000), but because these distinctions have been drawn quali-
tatively observers have frequently questioned their validity. Now, with
the advent of multinational epidemiological surveys across Europe,
cultural differences in drinking—and their impact on outcomes—have
been verified quantitatively. Cultures in which alcohol is most feared
to lead to problems and uncontrollable use—as a result of which
drinking is more regulated (e.g., limitations on outlets and times
where and when alcohol may be consumed)—paradoxically provoke
more binge drinking, negative social and psychological outcomes, and
addiction. The European Comparative Alcohol Study (ECAS), for example, found a negative correlation between the amount of alcohol
consumed within society and the prevalence of alcohol-related harm
in that society (Table 20.5). The United States has not been included
in these international surveys as yet, but the drinking data provided in
the National Survey on Drug Use and Health, particularly ethnic differences in rates of binge drinking, indicate that similar patterns pre-
vail among ethnic groups in this country (Table 20.6).

As a result, epidemiologists who participate in such surveys have
validated anthropological analyses, now supported by hard data:

In the northern countries, alcohol is described as a psychotropic
agent. It helps one to perform, maintains a Bacchic and heroic approach, and elates the self. It is used as an instrument to overcome
obstacles or to prove one's manliness. It has to do with the issue of
control and with its opposite—"discontrol" or transgression. (Allamani, 2002, p. 197)

In the southern countries, alcoholic beverages—mainly wine—are
drunk for their taste and smell, and are perceived as intimately
related to food, thus as an integral part of meals and family life.
Actually, wine tends to be considered as a food item. . . . It is traditionally consumed daily, at meals, in the family and other social
contexts. . . . Typically, Mediterranean people's drinking is still
characterized by relatively even weekly consumption, while in
northern cultures drinking is concentrated to rare occasions with
high intake per session. (Allamani, 2002, p. 200)

Thus, "safety" messages about the dangers of alcohol in temperance-
oriented cultures (mainly English-speaking and Scandinavian coun-

Table 20.5. Percentage of Males Drinking Daily, Binge Drinking, and Experiencing Drinking Harms, Selected European Countries

	Drinking Daily (%)	Binge Drinking per Drinking Occasion (%)	Experiencing Alcohol Harms (%)
Ireland	2	58	39
Sweden	3	32	36
Finland	4	29	47
United Kingdom	9	40	45
Germany	12	14	34
France	21	9	27
Italy	42	13	18

Source: Data from Ramstedt and Hope (2003), Hemström et al. (2002).

Table 20.6. Percentage of American Adults Who Binge Drink, by Ethnic/Racial Group

Ethnic/ Racial Group	Currently Drink* (%)	Binge† (%)	Percentage Who Binge/Percentage Drinkers
White	59	24	41
Black	44	24	55
Hispanic	47	27	57
Native American	48	29	60
Asian	41	14	34

Source: Data from SAMHSA (2003, Table 2.54B).
* Drank in the past month
† Binge = five or more drinks on a single occasion in the past month

tries) have unintended consequences reflected in the greater alcohol-related harm experienced in these countries (Hemström et al., 2002). Indeed, ECAS actually found a negative correlation between national levels of alcohol consumption and alcohol-related mortality due to cultural variations in drinking (Ramstedt, 2002). Addiction is not just a danger these cultures are dealing with; rather, these cultures are iatrogenically creating the conditions that enhance the likelihood of addiction.

The Treatment Implications of Disease Models of Addiction

Leading clinicians in the United States have fully embraced the disease model of addiction as reflecting the reality of their clinical practices and research (McClellan et al., 2000), and it is impossible for them to escape the limitations of their clinical perspective. Yet even within the clinical framework, the disease model has severe drawbacks. That is, a long tradition of psychological research has indicated the value of beliefs and treatments that enhance self-efficacy for overcoming problems. The disease model undercuts—denies the possibility of—such self-efficacy. Along with encouraging self-efficacy, psychological treatment models emphasize modifying environmental conditions and reinforcement in order to change behavior. What are the implications for outcomes of differences in treatment approaches?

One team of investigators has catalogued controlled clinical trials of alcoholism treatment over several decades (Miller et al., 2003). Their meta-analyses summarize the "cumulative evidence (of efficacy) score" for 48 popular modes of treatment (negative scores indicate relative ineffectiveness when compared in studies with other treatments—or no treatment). Table 20.7 lists selected results for effective (and ineffective) alcoholism therapies, with special reference to whether those therapies accept or reject the disease model of alcoholism.

Brief interventions (BIs), as their name indicates, are shorter in duration than conventional alcohol therapies. At their briefest, such an intervention can simply be an emergency care physician or general practitioner who notes a significant medical trauma or condition (e.g., poor liver function) and proceeds to instruct the patient to reduce or stop drinking. BIs are commonly used preventively in the absence of observed medical complications, where the physician just asks about the patient's drinking and may give advice based on the patient's answer. This first element of the BI is to provide feedback to the patient. In some BIs, providing this feedback and linking it to the patient's drinking and instructions to cut back or to quit comprise the entire intervention.

Motivational enhancement (ME) is a treatment geared to help people sort out their ambivalence about change, and to direct their own efforts to reducing their drinking. ME therapists assist people to change by, initially, asking open-ended questions about their drinking,

Table 20.7. Efficacy of Alcohol Treatments

Treatment	Cumulative Evidence Score
Brief intervention	390
Motivational enhancement	189
Community reinforcement approach	110
Self-change manual	110
Twelve-step facilitation	−82
Alcoholics Anonymous	−94
Confrontational counseling	−183
Psychotherapy	−207
General alcoholism counseling	−284
Education (tapes, etc.)	−443

Source: Data from Miller et al. (2003).

to assist clients in recognizing for themselves how their drinking is hurting them and violating values they hold. The key to ME is never to confront people—confrontational therapies have been shown to have little success and to produce other negative consequences.

The community reinforcement approach (CRA) is a package of behavioral techniques designed to encourage sobriety in more severely alcoholic (or dependent) patients than those typically treated with BIs and ME. CRA begins with a so-called functional analysis—that is, the when, where, and whys of the individual's drinking. Among the components of CRA are a job club (or vocational training), a leisure club (or recreational counseling) to direct the individual to nondrinking venues for entertainment, and relationship (or marital) therapy aimed at enhancing intimate relationships and ensuring that a spouse's behavior supports sobriety. If work, social time, and family or intimate life all reinforce the individual's ability to avoid drinking, his sobriety will be supported throughout his or her life space. Alcoholics are also trained in skills they must have to conduct themselves successfully in these situations.

These successful therapies are characterized by two principal underlying features: (1) each encourages people to take responsibility for their behavior—and to feel they can control these behaviors—and (2) alcoholism is not seen as a disease, but as a condition the individual can modify by changing behavior, environment, and effort. These results support a finding by Miller and colleagues in a prospective study of treatment outcomes. Two primary factors predicted relapse: "lack of coping skills and belief in the disease model of alcoholism" (Miller et al., 1996).

Conclusions

The disease model of addiction is disproved by basic evidence about the incidence and course of addictive substance use and is counterproductive in both the prevention and treatment of addiction. The key issues for addiction treatment in the twenty-first century are: the persistence of ingrained cultural beliefs in the face of scientific refutation and demonstrations that they are counterproductive, and whether new neuroscientific props will be used to support already demonstrably counterproductive attitudes and approaches to treating addiction (cf. McClellan et al., 2000).

REFERENCES

Allamani, A. 2002. Policy implications of the ECAS results: a southern European perspective. In T. Norstöm, ed., *Alcohol in Postwar Europe: Consumption, Drinking Patterns, Consequences and Policy Responses in 15 European Countries.* Stockholm: National Institute of Public Health.

Dawson, D.A. 1996. Correlates of past-year status among treated and untreated persons with former alcohol dependence: United States, 1992. *Alcoholism: Clinical and Experimental Research* 20:771–79.

Dawson, D.A., Grant, B.F., Stinson, F.S., Chou, P.S., Huang, B., and Ruan, W. J. 2005. Recovery from DSM-IV alcohol dependence, United States, 2001–2002. *Addiction* 100:281–92.

Erickson, P.G., Adlaf, E.M., Murray, G.F., and Smart, R.G. 1987. *The Steel Drug: Cocaine in Perspective.* Lexington, Mass.: Lexington.

Heath, D.B. 2000. *Drinking Occasions: Comparative Perspectives on Alcohol and Culture.* Philadelphia: Brunner/Mazel.

Hermström, O., Leifman, H., and Ramstedt, M. 2002. The ECAS survey on drinking patterns and alcohol-related problems. In T. Norström, ed., *Alcohol in Postwar Europe: Consumption, Drinking Patterns, Consequences and Policy Responses in 15 European Countries.* Stockholm: National Institute of Public Health.

McLellan, A.T., Lewis, D.C., O'Brien, C.P., and Kleber, H.D. 2000. Drug dependence, a chronic medical illness: Implications for treatment, insurance, and outcomes evaluation. *Journal of the American Medical Association* 284:1689–95.

Miller, W.R., Westerberg, V.S., Harris, R.J., and Tonigan, J. S. 1996. What predicts relapse? Prospective testing of antecedent models. *Addiction* 91 (Suppl.):S155–171.

Miller, W.R., Wilbourne, P.L., and Hettema, J.E. 2003. What works? A summary of alcohol treatment outcome research. In R. K. Hester and W. R. Miller, eds., *Handbook of Alcoholism Treatment Approaches: Effective Alternatives*, 3rd ed. Boston: Allyn and Bacon.

Peele, S. 1985. *The Meaning of Addiction: Compulsive Experience and Its Interpretation*. Lexington, Mass.: Lexington.

Peele, S., and DeGrandpre, R.J. 1998. Cocaine and the concept of addiction: environmental factors in drug compulsions. *Addiction Research* 6:235–63.

Ramstedt, M. 2002. Alcohol-related mortality in 15 European countries in the postwar period. In T. Norström, ed., *Alcohol in Postwar Europe: Consumption, Drinking Patterns, Consequences and Policy Responses in 15 European Countries*. Stockholm: National Institute of Public Health.

Ramstedt, M., and Hope, A. 2003. *The Irish Drinking Culture: Drinking and Drinking-Related Harm, a European Comparison*. Dublin, Ireland: Report for the Health Promotion Unit, Ministry of Health and Children.

Room, R. 1980. Treatment seeking populations and larger realities. In G. Edwards and M. Grant, eds., *Alcoholism Treatment in Transition*. London: Croom Helm.

Rudy, D. 1986. *Becoming Alcoholic: Alcoholics Anonymous and the Reality of Alcoholism*. Carbondale: Southern Illinois University Press.

Substance Abuse and Mental Health Services Administration. 2003. *Results from the 2002 National Survey on Drug Use and Health*. Rockville, Md.: U.S. Department of Health and Human Services.

21

Parsing the Future of Behavioral Intervention for Drug Abuse
Clinical Science and Policy

JESSE B. MILBY, PH.D.

Effective treatments for substance abuse include many behavioral interventions, including the management of policies and procedures in work sites, correctional systems, and other non-health-care settings. Although these interventions help many substance abusers, too many fail. The growing number of persons who are unemployed and chronically addicted may lead to change in social policy and programs if it becomes increasingly recognized that the status quo is not acceptable.

The potential for behavioral interventions using behavioral modification procedures termed "contingency management" (CM) was demonstrated by Cohen and colleagues (Cohen et al., 1971) with volunteer alcoholics who were allowed to drink in a controlled environment. Marked reductions in alcohol intake were observed during weeks when a contingency provided access to an enriched environment. Researchers soon demonstrated effectiveness of CM in communities. For example, controlled access to usual goods and services for skid row alcoholics reduced alcohol intake (verified by lower blood alcohol levels) and public drunkenness and increased employment. Similarly, take-home doses for methadone maintenance, contingent on abstinence from illicit drugs and achieving measurable therapeutic goals, improved treatment outcomes. A behavioral therapy involving CM was the first effective treatment for cocaine dependence (Higgins et al., 1991). At this writing, all effective treatments for cocaine dependence are behavioral interventions.

CM has also been incorporated in innovative interventions for dysfunctional and treatment-resistant populations. Abstinence CM procedures have been effective in programs that have trained participants in data entry skills and provided income and child care while greatly reducing or eliminating drug use among opioid-dependent pregnant women (Silverman et al., 2002). The effectiveness of abstinence contingent housing and work during CM behavioral day treatment for initiating and sustaining abstinence, employment, and housing has similarly been demonstrated among cocaine-dependent, homeless persons (Milby et al., 2003). Abstinence CM procedures are also reducing drug use and reinforcing other goal attainment for drug abuse offenders in drug court.

The effectiveness of these behavioral interventions for substance abuse argue for an optimistic view for their use by community service providers. Behavioral approaches to substance abuse treatment, however, have not been widely accepted or adopted as usual care. Instead they have been largely ignored by treatment providers. Why is this?

The prevailing model for substance abuse treatment is that of Alcoholics Anonymous (AA). Its wide acceptance among counselors and administrators has impeded adoption of effective behavioral interventions. Demonstrations of harm reduction with behavioral therapy via controlled drinking for some alcoholics, rather than absolute abstinence, contributed to rejection of these approaches by those who viewed absolute abstinence as the only legitimate treatment outcome. Also, with rising health care costs outpacing inflation, cost-cutting insurers appear reluctant to offer behavioral interventions in many areas of medicine (in addition to substance abuse) on their assumption that they are too costly.

There may yet, however, be reason for optimism with movement toward evidence-based practice, which could improve acceptance of effective behavioral interventions. Recently, for example, the AA movement has embraced research examination of its treatment procedures. Cost-effectiveness studies comparing usual care to effective behavioral interventions revealed the value of behavioral interventions to individuals and society. For example, the use of prize drawings and community provided incentives can be effective while reducing the costs of CM approaches for initiating and sustaining abstinence (Petry and Martin, 2002; Amass and Kamien, 2004). Counselor certification training exposes counselors to knowledge and skills needed to deliver effective behavioral interventions. Service providers increasingly accept that a master's degree is the minimum education requirement for substance abuse counselors

Future Challenges and Directions for Behavioral Interventions

A major challenge is to facilitate the diffusion of research-based treatment advances into the treatment system. Such facilitation may require increased support for demonstration and diffusion by the National Institutes of Health (NIH) and health care funders. Ideally, innovative service providers that are not dependent on NIH support could help disseminate advances in treatment more rapidly. These providers could adopt policies and procedures that reduce costs while extending the impact and acceptance of behavioral interventions. Internet-based interventions and counselor training could accelerate diffusion in the private sector and perhaps approach the critical mass needed for rapid widespread diffusion (Rogers, 2003).

The science foundation for treatment could also be enhanced by more active evaluation of the physiological effects of behavioral interventions. For example, effective interventions could be used to identify brain areas, via advanced imaging technology, that change in response to effective treatment. Responsive brain areas could then be targeted for focused interventions that use brain plasticity to improve brain-behavioral responsiveness. Identified areas could in turn become targets for medication development.

Behavioral interventions could also be incorporated effectively into programs that step up the treatment offering as is required by the patient ("stepped care"). Stepped care, combining effective interventions in a graded, sequential fashion, provides less intensive and less costly interventions to larger numbers of patients. For those who do not respond to initial treatment, care is stepped up to more intensive interventions. Stepped care could combine behavioral interventions with other effective interventions like motivational interviewing or pharmacotherapies, such as disulfiram, methadone, or naltrexone. An example of stepped care is found in a recent study of treatment for cocaine-dependent homeless persons in which abstinence contingent housing and vocational intervention were used as a first step (Milby et al., 2005). In this randomized controlled trial, an intensive CM behavioral day treatment using vouchers was employed as a second step comparison. High initial and sustained abstinence for both groups—more than 55 percent—was attained at six months, but longer-term abstinence outcomes at 12 and 18 months favored stepped-up care. Future adaptations could be designed to refer patients who do not respond to initial care to CM behavioral day treatment. Stepped care for treatment-resistant patients is exemplified in the work of Silverman and colleagues, in which voucher reinforcement for cocaine abstinence in methadone-treated opioid-dependent patients was utilized (Silverman et al., 1999). Magnitude of reinforcement (i.e., steps) was a critical determinant of effectiveness. Programs designed to include stepped care for future services could identify at admission the most severely addicted, unemployed patients for whom previous treatment had failed. Instead of more failed treatment episodes these patients could be referred to interventions using unemployment and disability benefits for contingent compensation in a therapeutic work place modeled after Silverman and colleagues (2002).

The U.S. population includes growing numbers of unemployed people who are chronically addicted. Many are living in poverty and often resort to illegal activities to support their habit and their families. Society incurs considerable welfare costs providing health care, unemployment benefits, and substance abuse services, as well as the costs of the criminal justice system and of crime itself. Yet interventions for these individuals frequently fail. Their growing numbers should be a siren call for change in social policy that could substantially improve not only the lives of individuals but also societal cost-benefit ratios.

A well-designed, publicly supported treatment system that combined training, work, and substance abuse intervention could address these interdependent domains in a coordinated and integrated manner. Social welfare benefits could be made contingent on participation and reduced, if not eliminated, illicit drug use, until the patient obtains private sector employment. For those who fail to obtain private sector employment, continued public benefits could be contingent on reduced or eliminated drug abuse, community service work, or training to prepare for private sector employment. Such a system would benefit society from community services and public works' projects similar to those contributed by the Depression-era Civilian Conservation Corps. It would keep those receiving benefits in a program that both monitors and reinforces self-control over drug abuse.

Such a program would require strong public support and funding, but it has the potential to contribute to public health while reducing societal costs by reducing expenditures for health care, adjudication, and incarceration. A logical administrative home for such a program would be to subsume it under the federal workfare program, as detailed by Frison and Milby (2000).

A continuum of applied behavior change principles could extend from full societal support of programs and policies to use well-established behavior change principles within existing programs to improve their effectiveness. Diffusion of effective behavioral interventions could be aided by innovators who increase effectiveness or reduce costs. Finally, the concept that effective and innovative service providers deserve greater reward (including financial compensation) is recognized in many areas of our society, including many medical specialties. Sadly, it does not seem to be recognized in addiction treatment. Policymakers who dare to find ways to share financial benefits of reduced substance abuse with the providers that make such contributions to health could also contribute to increased innovation, diffusion of innovations, and improved public health.

ACKNOWLEDGMENTS

This chapter was completed while the author was Visiting Professor at the Johns Hopkins University Center for Learning and Health and the Behavioral Pharmacology Research Unit. Ideas contained here were inspired and exchanged with Kenneth Silverman, Ph.D.; Conrad Wong, Ph.D.; Roland Griffiths, Ph.D.; Maxine Stitzer, Ph.D.; George Bigelow, Ph.D.; Eric Strain, M.D.; Van King, M.D.; Robert Brooner, Ph.D.; and many other psychiatrist colleagues at the Department of Psychiatry luncheon meetings, colloquia, seminars, and informal discussions. To these colleagues and Johns Hopkins University, I am deeply grateful for the opportunity to study with and learn from them during the academic year 2004–2005. They, however, bear no responsibility for the ideas conveyed or ignored here.

REFERENCES

Amass, L., and Kamien, J. R. 2004. A tale of two cities: financing two voucher programs for substance abusers through donations. *Experimental and Clinical Psychopharmacology* 12(2):147–55.

Cohen, M., Liebson, I., Faillace, L. A., and Allen, R. P. 1971. Moderate drinking by chronic alcoholics. *Journal of Nervous and Mental Disease* 153:434–44.

Frison, S., and Milby, J. B. 2004. Intervening through the social welfare system: a proposed contingency management program with implications for workfare planning. In W. Miller and C. Weisner, eds., *Addressing Addictions through Health and Social Systems*. New York: Plenum Press.

Higgins, S. T., Delaney, D. D., Budney, A. J., Bickel, W. K., Hughes J. R., Foerg, F., and Fenwick, J. W. 1991. A behavioral approach to achieving initial cocaine abstinence. *American Journal of Psychiatry* 148:1218–24.

Milby, J. B., Schumacher, J. E., Wallace, D., Freedman, M. J., Kertesz, S., Vikinsalo, M., and Vuchinich, R. E. 2005. CM for housing and work performance are sufficient to establish sustained abstinence in homeless substance abusers. Presented at the College on Problems of Drug Dependence, June 21, Orlando, Fla.

Milby, J. B., Schumacher, J. E., Wallace, D., Frison, S., McNamara, C., Usdan, S., and Michael, M. 2003. Day treatment with contingency management for cocaine abuse in homeless persons: 12-month follow-up. *Journal of Consulting and Clinical Psychology* 71:619–21.

Petry, N. M., and Martin, B. 2002. Low-cost contingency management for treating cocaine- and opioid-abusing methadone patients. *Journal of Consulting and Clinical Psychology* 70:398–405.

Rogers, E. M. 2003. *Diffusion of Innovations,* 5th ed. New York: Free Press.

Silverman, K., Chutuape, M. A., Bigelow, G. E., and Stitzer, M. L. 1999. Voucher-based reinforcement of cocaine abstinence in treatment-resistant methadone patients: effects of reinforcement magnitude. *Psychopharmacology* 146:128–38.

Silverman, K., Svikis, D., Wong, C.J., Hampton, J., Stitzer M. L., and Bigelow, G. E. 2002. A reinforcement-based therapeutic workplace for the treatment of drug abuse: three year abstinence outcomes. *Experimental and Clinical Psychopharmacology* 10:228–40.

22

Protecting Patient Confidentiality in Alcohol and Drug Treatment

PAUL N. SAMUELS, J.D.

The publication in 2003 of the final Privacy Rule under the federal Health Insurance Portability and Accountability Act (HIPAA), confidentiality rules that govern the vast majority of health care providers in the United States, shone a national spotlight on an issue that has been of prime importance to the alcohol and drug service provider community for three decades. Confidentiality has been a key feature of alcohol and drug treatment and prevention programs, in significant part because their patients often face two major risks that most consumers of health services do not have to worry about: discrimination and arrest. HIPAA and alcohol and drug confidentiality laws enacted in the early 1970s are similar in many respects, but their differences are important and the result of those special risks. Understanding those differences is critical both to protecting patients' rights and the viability of the system for delivering alcohol and drug services and charting a course for improving how our nation addresses addiction and the millions of Americans who are addicted or are in recovery.

In the early 1970s, the federal government enacted laws to guarantee the strict confidentiality of information about persons receiving alcohol and drug prevention and treatment services, one dealing with patient records and information involving alcohol abuse and the other drug abuse. Both statutes established the same confidentiality and disclosure rules; in 1992 Congress consolidated them into one law (at 42 U.S.C. §290dd-2). These statutes have always been implemented by a single set of federal regulations, which were first issued in 1975 and revised in 1987. The U.S. Department of Health and Human Services (HHS) is the federal agency that issued and has primary responsibility for interpreting the regulations.

The drug and alcohol confidentiality regulations, codified in 42 C.F.R. Part 2, require agencies and professionals providing federally assisted alcohol and drug services to obtain the written consent of the patient in most circumstances before disclosures about diagnosis, referral, counseling, or other services can be made. Disclosures can be made by an alcohol or drug program without written consent of the patient only if they meet the criteria of the few narrowly drawn exceptions to the consent requirement.[1]

When passed in 1996, HIPAA contemplated that Congress would then enact a set of specific requirements for health care providers to maintain the confidentiality of their records but required HHS to promulgate regulations if Congress failed to act. When Congress was unable to agree on privacy rules, HHS issued regulations on April 14, 2003, that protect the privacy of health care information held by the vast majority of health care providers, health plans, and health care clearing houses (45 C.F.R. 160, 164). Although HIPAA applies only to agencies that transmit information electronically, that covers most of the nation's health care provider system.

The HIPAA Privacy Rule, like 42 C.F.R. Part 2 on which it was largely patterned, requires in many circumstances that patients sign a specific authorization form before a health care agency can make disclosures about the patient. Indeed, both sets of rules address many of the same issues in largely the same ways, establishing standards for the maintenance, use, and disclosure of health information, including what must be done before a disclosure of confidential information can be made, the manner in which the information may be disclosed, and to whom it may be disclosed.

There are, however, several differences between HIPAA and 42 C.F.R. Part 2 that have significant practical and public policy implications. Two of the most important differences concern when and how disclosures can be made to law enforcement and to insurance companies and other private and public payers.

The HIPAA Privacy Rule allows disclosures to law enforcement agencies and for judicial proceedings without written patient consent or any other authorization.[2] In contrast, 42 C.F.R. Part 2 prohibits disclosures to law enforcement and courts unless patients sign a consent form, and if the disclosure sought is for the purpose of investigating or prosecuting the patient even a signed consent form is insufficient; a court must first issue a special order after holding a hearing and making findings that the disclosure is so important that it outweighs the need to maintain confidentiality of alcohol and drug patient records.

The critical importance of these confidentiality protections to the viability of our nation's alcohol and drug treatment and prevention system cannot be overstated. What Congress recognized when it first enacted the confidentiality laws three decades ago remains just as true today: if drug and alcohol treatment records are readily available to law enforcement officials and courts without limitation or judicial oversight, few people would be willing to enter treatment. Who would voluntarily enroll in treatment if they knew that their treatment records would be available on request to any police officer or district attorney who might want to arrest and prosecute them? Or to any spouse who was looking for damaging information to introduce into evidence in a custody or divorce case?

Preventing exactly these kinds of scenarios may be the principal reason why the drug and alcohol confidentiality rules were enacted in the first place. The HIPAA Privacy Rule, however, grew out of a general concern that lack of uniform federal confidentiality rules for health care records led to widespread violations of medical privacy and inconsistent rules from one state to the next. Disclosures to law enforcement or courts were barely on the radar screen, if at all, and were left unregulated.

The HIPAA Privacy Rule also permits a patient's medical information to be disclosed for payment purposes without patient consent,[3] but 42 C.F.R. Part 2 requires the patient's written consent for disclosures to insurance companies, Medicaid, Medicare, or any other payer and also before redisclosure of that information to anyone else, including an employer who may be paying for the coverage. Among other benefits, this requirement protects people receiving drug and alcohol treatment from discrimination. Some insurance companies refuse to issue individual insurance policies to people in recovery from addiction, and some employers fire or refuse to hire people in recovery. For example, a poll conducted for Faces and Voices of Recovery August 2–22, 2001, by Peter Hart and Associates found that 24 percent of people in recovery report suffering discrimination in insurance or employment. The requirement that the patient sign a consent form before disclosures can be made for payment enables those receiving services to consider such possible risks before deciding whether to authorize the disclosure. Some patients who can afford it decide to pay for treatment out of pocket to avoid the potential for future discrimination.

From time to time some who work in the alcohol and drug treatment field lament the need for the heightened confidentiality protections afforded by 42 C.F.R. Part 2 and wonder whether eliminating them would help dispel the stigma, prejudice, and discrimination against people in recovery still too rampant in our nation, but 42 C.F.R. Part 2 is the prophylactic response to discrimination and overzealous prosecution, not the cause. We all look forward to the day when those problems have disappeared, but until it arrives, 42 C.F.R. Part 2 remains an indispensable bulwark against intrusion that ensures that those who need drug and alcohol services will step forward to obtain them without fear.

ACKNOWLEDGMENT

This chapter relies heavily on *Confidentiality and Communication: A Guide to the Federal Drug and Alcohol Confidentiality Law and HIPAA* (2003) by the Legal Action Center.

NOTES

1. These include (1) internal communications necessary to provision of services can be made within an agency; (2) information can be disclosed that does not identify a patient such as aggregate data; (3) qualified personnel may obtain information in a medical emergency; (4) those covered by state child abuse and neglect mandatory reporting laws can (and must) make those reports; (5) special agreements can be signed with those who provide ongoing services to the program; (6) qualified researchers, auditors, and evaluators can obtain information but must abide by strict limits on use and disclosure; (7) programs can report and obtain the assistance of law enforcement if a crime is committed or threatened on the program's premises or against program personnel; and (8) a court can issue a special order authorizing disclosures after following a strict set of standards and procedural safeguards.

2. The HIPAA Privacy Rule requires the recipient of a subpoena, discovery request, or other lawful process to be assured or itself ensure that reasonable efforts have been made either (1) to ensure that the individual(s) who are the subject of the information have been notified of the request so

they could object or (2) to secure a qualified protective order for the information. See 45 CFR 164.512(e). But, unlike 42 CFR Part 2, HIPAA creates no standards limiting when disclosures can be made in a court proceeding.

3. 45 C.F.R. §§ 164.502(a), 164.506(c).

REFERENCES

Legal Action Center. 2003. *Confidentiality and Communication: A Guide to the Federal Drug & Alcohol Confidentiality Law and HIPAA.* New York: Legal Action Center.

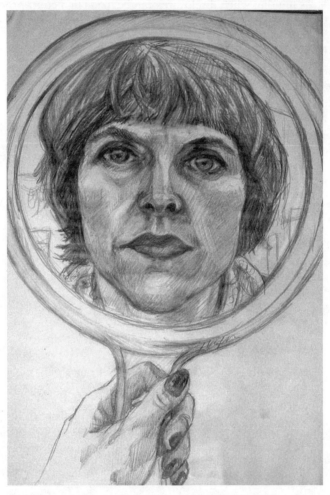

(Self) Portrait of an Alcoholic, by Lizabeth Kelly Lyles

23

Deterring Sales and Marketing of Alcohol to Youth
The Role of Litigation

ALEXANDER C. WAGENAAR, PH.D.

The single most effective teen alcohol prevention effort in the past half-century has been the passage of laws in all 50 U.S. states prohibiting sales to, or purchase and consumption of alcoholic beverages by, anyone younger than 21 years. These laws have produced long-term reductions in teen drinking of about 15 percent and reduced alcohol-related injuries and deaths by 10–20 percent (see Wagenaar and Toomey [2002] for a review of more than 100 studies). At least 20,000 people are alive today who would have been killed as teenagers had we not passed age-21 laws in the 1970s and early 1980s (National Highway Traffic Safety Administration, 2003).

These substantial public health and safety benefits were obtained even though efforts to publicize and enforce the law have been minimal, especially in the early years after passage of the age-21 laws. Estimates reveal that only two in 1,000 occasions of drinking by underage youth result in an arrest or citation of the young drinker, and only five in 100,000 result in any enforcement action taken against the bar or liquor store that sold the alcohol illegally to underage patrons (Wagenaar and Wolfson, 1994). And in many communities, half or more of alcohol retailers sell alcohol to youth without requesting age identification, despite laws prohibiting such sales (Preusser and Williams, 1992; Forster et al., 1994; Wagenaar et al., 1996; Grube, 1997; Freisthler et al., 2003). As a result of such easy access to alcohol, recent data show that 48 percent of high school seniors have drunk al-

Table 23.1. Lawsuits on Marketing Alcohol to Youth

Jurisdiction	Date Filed	Case Name	Status
California	02/03/04	*Goodwin v. Anheuser-Busch Co. & Miller Brewing Co.*	Judgment on the pleadings for defendants 01/27/05. On appeal.
Colorado	12/03/03	*Kreft v. Zima Beverage Co., et al.*	Dismissed with prejudice; plaintiff to pay defendants' attorneys' fees. On appeal.
District of Columbia	11/14/03	*Hakki v. Zima Beverage Co., et al.*	Pending trial in district court
Florida	03/22/04	*Badillo, et al. v. Playboy Entertainment, Anheuser-Busch, et al.*	Pending trial in state court (plaintiffs motion for preliminary injunction denied, 04/16/04)
Florida	03/30/05	*Kornhauzer v. Adolph Coors Co., et al.*	Pending trial in state court
Michigan	03/30/05	*Alston v. Advanced Brands & Importing Co., et al.*	Pending trial in state court
North Carolina	01/13/04	*Wilson v. Zima Beverage Co., et al.*	Pending trial in federal court
Nevada	04/14/04	*Pisco v. Coors Brewing Co., et al.*	Dismissed 06/09/04
New York	02/16/05	*Sciocchetti v. Advanced Brands & Importing Co., et al.*	Pending trial in state court
Ohio	04/30/04	*Eisenberg v. Anheuser-Busch, Inc., et al.*	Pending trial in federal court
Ohio	06/09/04	*Tully v. Anheuser-Busch, Inc., et al.*	Pending trial in federal court
Wisconsin	02/27/05	*Tomberlin v. Adolph Coors, et al.*	Pending trial in state court

cohol in the past month and 33 percent have consumed five or more drinks at a time—in other words, have gotten drunk—in the past 30 days (Johnston et al., 2005). In short, the age-21 legal drinking age has significantly reduced teen drinking and alcohol-related deaths, but modest implementation and enforcement means youth still can obtain alcohol easily. Underage drinkers currently consume 10–20 percent of all alcohol sold in the United States, representing a market of more than $15 billion per year (Foster et al., 2003; Institute of Medicine, 2004).

At the most basic level, laws compel healthy, safe, and socially beneficial behaviors and prohibit unhealthy, dangerous, and socially deleterious behaviors by shaping incentives (rewards) and deterrents (punishments). In the case of alcohol, extremely dangerous behaviors, such as driving while intoxicated, are directly prohibited, while a system of many laws and regulations shape allowable ways alcohol can be produced, marketed, distributed, and sold. Such laws and regulations have significant effects on how much people drink and the levels of alcohol-related harm a community experiences (Toomey and Wagenaar, 1999; Babor et al., 2003).

Litigation—that is, the use of the courts to enforce an obligation (as opposed to convict a person of a criminal offense)—is a tool that can complement criminal law to promote public health. Those who manufacture, distribute, or sell alcoholic beverages have an obligation to not entice or promote teen alcohol use, to not market alcohol to teens, and to take reasonable actions to prevent sales to anyone younger than 21. Since the 1990s, individuals and organizations have filed a number of lawsuits to enforce that obligation, given (1) the substantial proportion of the alcohol market accounted for by illegal sales; (2) advertising and promotion on television, in magazines, and at spring break and sports/music venues with large proportions of the audience under age 21; and (3) the promotion of "alcopop" products with sweet flavors that are appealing to youth and new drinkers (Smeaton et al., 1998; Leeming et al., 2002; Garfield et al., 2003; Jernigan et al., 2004). Recent lawsuits are mostly class action cases against alcohol producers arguing that the producers' advertising and marketing practices illegally target underage youth (Table 23.1). The lawsuits seek monetary awards to compensate for the resulting harm, injunctive relief to halt the illegal marketing, and punitive damages.

Litigation serves two functions when it recognizes failures to meet obligations: it provides financial *compensation* to individuals for harms experienced and, of greatest interest for the present analysis, it serves to *prevent* future harm (Christoffel and Teret, 1991). Litigation has five main mechanisms for achieving preventive effects. First, the process of developing evidence for a lawsuit (*discovery*) brings to light noxious behaviors and practices of the defendant, such as particularly egregious and blatant practices inducing youth to drink. For example, attorneys for the plaintiff (the party starting the lawsuit) typically request and obtain internal documents and records of the defendant that are directly relevant to the case. Second, *publicity* of the lawsuit and evidence revealed in it can both be unfavorable to the defendant and thus serve as a deterrent and more broadly put teen drinking issues on the agenda of the media, the public, and policymakers. Publicity can also lead to longer-term normative changes regarding acceptable patterns of alcohol sales and use. Third, court orders for addressing the problem (*injunctive relief*) require the defendant to cease and desist from marketing and advertising campaigns that target minors. Fourth, payment of *damages and fees*, both actual (e.g., what the damage actually cost those affected) and, especially, punitive (e.g., what the court and jury consider appropriate punishment given the circumstances of the case). Fifth, *disgorgement* acts as a deterrent—that is, compelling alcohol companies to return the profits gained from illegal sales to minors ("ill-gotten" profits). Damages and disgorgement also can result in increased retail prices of alcohol as companies adjust to cover these costs. Higher prices are known to reduce alcohol consumption and associated health and social problems (Coate and Grossman, 1988; Chesson et al., 2000; Adrian et al., 2001; Cook and Moore, 2002; Farrell et al., 2003).

The use of litigation to address the marketing and sales of alcohol to teens is often compared to the experience with litigation to address the marketing and sales of tobacco to youth. There are many parallels, but also some important differences. One difference is the early evolutionary stage of alcohol suits. Lawsuits against alcohol companies are just now being initiated, with only a dozen suits pending or recently completed (Table 23.1). Litigation against tobacco companies was first initiated almost a half century ago, with the number of pending cases increasing gradually to approximately 600 by the late 1990s and increasing markedly to more than 3,000 in the early 2000s (Jacobson and Soliman, 2002). Early cases in a new area of law often are unsuccessful as various legal theories are tested in a social environment in which concerns about the health effects of the product at issue are as yet only modest. Thus, it is unlikely that in the United States there will be numerous successful cases with substantial injunctive and financial penalties against alcohol companies in the near future. On the other hand, precedents of the tobacco litigation likely will significantly shorten the evolutionary history of such suits in the case of alcohol.

Finally, what is the evidence that successful litigation achieves prevention of harm? Unfortunately, the debate about the *effectiveness* of litigation is colored by controversy about the *appropriateness* of litigation, a controversy rooted in vested interests and competing political philosophies (e.g., free enterprise capitalism, paternalism/libertarianism, roles of legislative vs. judicial branches of government). Nevertheless, studies of the effects of the tobacco litigation of the late 1990s are already emerging, with evidence accumulating that marketing changed, prices increased, and consumption declined (Keeler et al., 2004). Most scientists and legal analysts observing recent experience with tobacco litigation agree that litigation has substantially advanced the prevention of tobacco-related harm, though it is also clear that legislating and actively implementing and enforcing policies are also important for effective tobacco control (Jacobson and Warner, 1999; Jacobson and Soliman, 2002; Daynard, 2003). For alcohol control, we already know that numerous legislated policies and regulations that control when, where, how and to whom alcohol is sold are effective in reducing alcohol-related harm, and at this early stage it appears that litigation is likely to be an important complement.

REFERENCES

Adrian, M., Ferguson, B.S., and Her, M. 2001. Can alcohol price policies be used to reduce drunk driving? Evidence from Canada. *Substance Use and Misuse* 36 (13):1923–57.

Babor, T., Caetano, R., Casswell, S., Edwards, G., Giesbrecht, N., Graham, K., Grube, J., Gruenewald, P., Hill, L., Holder, H., Homel, R., Osterberg, E., Rehm, R., Room, R., and Rossow, I. 2003. *Alcohol: No Ordinary Commodity.* New York: Oxford University Press.

Chesson, H., Harrison, P., and Kassler, W. J. 2000. Sex under the influence: the effect of alcohol policy on sexually transmitted disease rates in the United States. *Journal of Law and Economics* 43 (1):215–38.

Christoffel, J. D., and Teret, J. D. 1991. Epidemiology and the law: courts and confidence intervals. *Public Health and the Law* 81 (12):1661–66.

Coate, D., and Grossman, M. 1988. Effects of alcoholic beverage prices and legal drinking ages on youth alcohol use. *Journal of Law and Economics* 31 (1):145–71.

Cook, P. J., and Moore, M. J. 2002. The economics of alcohol abuse and alcohol-control policies. *Drugs, Economics and Policy* 21(2):120–33.

Daynard, R. 2003. Why tobacco litigation? *Tobacco Control* 12:1–2.

Farrell, S., Manning, W. G., and Finch, M. D. 2003. Alcohol dependence and the price of alcoholic beverages. *Journal of Health Economics* 22:117–47.

Foster, S. E., Vaughn, R. D., Foster, W. H., and Califano, J. A. 2003. Alcohol consumption and expenditures for underage drinking and adult excessive drinking. *JAMA* 289 (8):989–95.

Forster, J. L., McGovern, P. G., Wagenaar, A. C., Wolfson, M., Perry, C. L., and Anstine, P. S. 1994. The ability of young people to purchase alcohol without age identification in northeastern Minnesota, USA. *Addiction* 89:699–705.

Freisthler, B., Greenwald, P. J., Freno, A. J., and Lee, J. 2003. Evaluating alcohol access and the alcohol environment in neighborhood areas. *Alcoholism: Clinical and Experimental Research* 276 (3):477–84.

Garfield, C. F., Chung, P. J., and Rathouy, P. J. 2003. Alcohol advertising in magazines and adolescent readership. *JAMA* 289 (18):2424–29.

Grube, J. W. 1997. Preventing sales of alcohol to minors: results from a community trial. *Addiction* 92 (S2):5251–60.

Institute of Medicine. 2004. *Reducing Underage Drinking: A Collective Responsibility*, edited by R. J. Bonnie and M. E. O'Connell. Washington, D.C.: National Academies Press.

Jacobson, P. D., and Soliman, S. 2002. Litigation as public health policy: theory or reality? *Journal of Law, Medicine & Ethics* 30:224–38.

Jacobson, P. D., and Warner, K. E. 1999. Litigation and public health policy: the case of tobacco control. *Journal of Health Politics, Policy and Law* 24:769–804.

Jernigan, D. H., Ostroff, J., Ross, C., and O'Hara, J. A. 2004. Sex differences in adolescent exposure to alcohol advertising in magazines. *Archives of Pediatric and Adolescent Medicine* 158:629–34.

Johnston, L. D., O'Malley, P. M., and Bachman, J. G. 2005. *Monitoring the Future: National Results on Adolescent Drug Use: Overview of Key Findings, 2004*. NIH publication no. 05-5726. Bethesda, Md.: National Institute on Drug Abuse.

Keeler, T. E., Hu, T., Ong, M., and Sung, H. 2004. The US National Tobacco Settlement: the effects of advertising and price changes on cigarette consumption. *Applied Economics* 36:1623–29.

Leeming, D., Harley, M., and Lyttle, S. 2002. Young people's images of cigarettes, alcohol and drugs. *Drugs-Education Prevention and Policy* 9(2):169–85.

National Highway Traffic Safety Administration. 2003. *Traffic Safety Facts 2002: Young Drivers*. DOT HS 809 619. Washington, D.C.: Department of Transportation.

Preusser, D. F., and Williams, A. F. 1992. Sales of alcohol to underage purchasers in three New York counties and Washington D.C. *Journal of Public Health Policy* 13:306–17.

Smeaton, G. L., Josiam, B. M., and Dietrich, I. C. 1998. College students' binge drinking at a beachfront destination during spring break. *Journal of American College Health* 46 (6):247–54.

Toomey, T. L., and Wagenaar, A. C. 1999. Policy options for prevention: the case of alcohol. *Journal of Public Health Policy* 20 (2):192–213.

Wagenaar, A. C., and Toomey, T. L. 2002. Effects of minimum drinking age laws: review and analyses of the literature. *Journal of Studies on Alcohol* Suppl. 14:206–25.

Wagenaar, A. C., and Wolfson, M. 1994. Enforcement of the legal minimum drinking age in the United States. *Journal of Public Health Policy* 15 (1):37–53.

Wagenaar, A. C., Toomey, T. L., Murray, D. M., Short, B. J., Wolfson, M., Jones-Webb, R. 1996. Sources of alcohol for underage drinkers. *Journal of Studies on Alcohol* 57:325–33.

24

How Social Policy Can Foster Advances in the Treatment of Addiction
Tobacco Smoke Pollution and the Hospitality Industry as an Example

JAMES L. REPACE, M.SC.

Should government protect workers from harmful working conditions that could cause serious injury to their health and even loss of life? Should the public be protected from exposure to harmful agents in air, water, and food? Should these protections proceed despite potential adverse economic consequences for affected industries? In the United States, the answer has been "yes." Federal laws—such as the Federal Hazardous Substance Act, the Consumer Product Safety Act, the Fair Packaging and Labeling Act, the Controlled Substances Act, the Toxic Substances Control Act, the Pure Food and Drug Act, the Clean Air Act, the Clean Water Act, and the Occupational Safety and Health Act—are intended to prevent illness and death as a result of public or occupational exposures to harmful substances in air, water, and food and are enforced by such regulatory bodies as the Environmental Protection Agency (EPA), the Occupational Safety and Health Administration (OSHA), and the Food and Drug Administration.

Secondhand smoke should be a strong candidate for federal regulation, because it has been condemned as a grave health hazard by every U.S. occupational health, environmental health, and public health authority since 1986. Smoking has been prohibited in many federal workplaces and on commercial aircraft for more than *two decades*. Nevertheless, because of intense congressional pressure, instigated by the powerful tobacco lobby, U.S. regulatory agencies have been discouraged from protecting private sector workers and the general public, and there is no legal authority by which the toxic emissions of tobacco products can be regulated. Because nonindustrial indoor air pollution remains largely unregulated, health departments often lack a legal mandate for controlling secondhand smoke, and legislatures at the state, county, and city level have become the battlegrounds, especially over smoking bans in the hospitality industry.

Arguments by businesses against regulation have focused on predictions of economic harm if smoking is banned in restaurants and bars, claims that ventilation or air cleaning, often in conjunction with designated smoking areas, provide acceptable alternatives to smoking bans, and assertions that secondhand smoke poses a far lower exposure to air pollution than air pollution from traffic. None of these arguments is actually supported by data.

Economics

In essence, the "economic impact" argument holds that the hospitality industry will incur economic losses as a result of smoke-free workplace laws, but if it is true that smokers will simply avoid patronizing smoke-free hospitality venues, by the same token why wouldn't it be true that nonsmokers would similarly avoid smoky venues? And, if *that* is true, has this industry already suffered a loss of trade among the majority of its potential customers, because nonsmokers outnumber smokers by four or five to one? There is a plethora of published data showing that smoking bans do not lead to economic losses for the hospitality industry (Novick, 1999; California Department of Health Services, Tobacco Control Section, 2001; Mandel et al., 2005). It is worth looking closely at some salient examples.

The Irish Experience

What has been the outcome of the 2004 Irish ban on workplace smoking? Compliance has been 93 percent in pubs and restaurants. Despite the prophets of doom, Irish pubs are not closing down in droves, and since the ban went into effect several pubs have been sold for record amounts. Ninety-eight percent of Irish people surveyed believe that workplaces are healthier. Air quality in pubs has improved dramatically since the smoke-free law went into effect. Bar sales declined in volume by 4.4 percent in 2004, compared to a decline of 4.2 percent for the previous year. Economic analysts suggest that this continuing downward trend is due to a number of factors beyond the smoking ban itself, including high prices, changing lifestyles, and shifting demographic patterns. At the same time, however, there is evidence that food sales have increased, reflecting a shift in the general public's attitude toward the pub being regarded as a suitable place to have a meal rather than simply a venue to socialize around alcohol. The data show a decline in bar sales of 2.4 percent between the end of 2003 and 2004. Nonetheless, the numbers of workers employed in the sector at the end of 2004 exceeded those employed in 2002 by 0.6 percent.

The New York City Experience

When the Smoke Free Air Act took effect on March 30, 2003, questions were raised about how the law would affect New York City's restaurants and bars. Would the law hurt business? Would some establishments have to lay off workers or close? One year later, the city's bar and restaurant industry was thriving and its workers were breathing cleaner, safer air. Since the law was enacted, 97 percent of restaurants and bars have become smoke free. Business receipts for restaurants and bars have increased—2004 tax receipts increased 8.7 percent compared to 2003 levels; employment in the hospitality sector has added 10,000 jobs (about 2,800 seasonally adjusted jobs); and the number of new liquor licenses issued has grown—all signs that New York City bars and restaurants are prospering. The vast majority of New Yorkers support the law and say they are more likely to patronize bars and restaurants now that they are smoke free. Air quality in bars and restaurants has improved dramatically: levels of cotinine, a by-product of tobacco, decreased by 85 percent in nonsmoking workers in bars and restaurants, and 150,000 fewer New Yorkers are exposed to secondhand smoke on the job (New York City Department of Finance et al., 2004).

The California Experience

In 2001, 86 percent of California nonsmokers and 59 percent of California smokers strongly agreed that they prefer to eat in restaurants that are smoke free. The establishment of smoke-free bars and taverns in California was associated with improvements in the respiratory health of bartenders but had no negative effect on the profitability of restaurants and bars. Despite tobacco industry arguments to the contrary, tax data demonstrate that smoking bans in restaurants and bars did not adversely impact revenues (California Department of Health Services, Tobacco Control Section, 2004).

The Massachusetts Experience

According to a Harvard University study, during the first six months of Massachusetts's statewide smoking ban, sales and employment at Massachusetts restaurants and bars grew slightly, disproving predictions that the prohibition would inflict serious damage on the hospitality industry. This is not surprising. In 1995–1996, Biener and Fitzgerald at the University of Massachusetts (Boston) surveyed a representative sample of 4,929 Massachusetts adults to assess who avoids smoky restaurants and bars, and why (Biener and Fitzgerald, 1999). The adult population of Massachusetts (18 years) was 4.5 million, 3.7 million of whom were nonsmokers and 800,000 of whom were smokers. Biener and colleagues found that 76 percent of the nonsmokers were bothered by tobacco smoke and that 46 percent of nonsmokers sampled reported that they avoided smoky places because of offensive odors or health worries. The study estimated that 515,405 adult nonsmokers avoided smoky restaurants and 364,400 nonsmokers avoided bars because of secondhand smoke. This means that 880,000 nonsmokers avoided smoky restaurants and bars—80,000 persons more than the total number of all adult smokers. As part of the study, analysts from the Harvard School of Public Health tested the air in 27 bars and restaurants both before and after the ban went into effect in July 2004. They found that toxins plummeted by 93 percent once smoking was banished.

Most economic arguments have focused on predicted costs to businesses of smoking bans and overlook the costs to workers from secondhand smoke. Workers bear the brunt of the diseases of secondhand smoke, and OSHA estimates that between 2,200 and 13,700 U.S. workers die annually directly from exposure to secondhand smoke. Repace and colleagues estimated 4,400 worker deaths per year from lung cancer and heart disease due to passive smoking at a worker exposure prevalence of 28 percent (Repace et al., 1998). Based on the U.S. EPA estimate of the value of a statistical life of $4.8 million (U.S. EPA, 1997), those 4,400 deaths represented a societal cost of $21 billion per year. These statistics are never quoted by opponents of smoking bans.

Some have argued that workers who are concerned for their health can simply choose to work elsewhere. Presumably, those workers who are well informed about the hazards of passive smoking *and* who have alternatives have already made this choice. Moreover, this argument avoids discussion of employers' common-law obligations to maintain a safe and healthy workplace. If the hospitality industry does incur economic losses as a result of smoke-free workplace laws, should it, alone among all other industries, be exempt from providing a safe and healthy workplace to profit from facilitating an addiction that will cause the premature deaths of most of its smoking patrons?

Ventilation

It has also been argued that workplaces can be made safe for workers and the public simply by application of ventilation or air cleaning. The available data, however, clearly show that ventilation or air cleaning cannot possibly provide air that is safe to breathe in the presence of smoking (Repace, 2004, 2005).

In 1994, OSHA, a division of the U.S. Department of Labor, stated in a proposed rule, "The carcinogenicity of environmental tobacco smoke discounts the use of general ventilation as an engineering control for this contaminant" and would result in "significant risk of material impairment of health to nonsmoking workers." OSHA proposed that all workplaces be made smoke free for the protection of workers. In 2005, the American Society of Heating, Refrigerating, and Air-conditioning Engineers (ASHRAE) Environmental Tobacco Smoke (ETS) Position Document issued a position paper stating that,

> Although complete separation and isolation of smoking rooms can control ETS exposure in non-smoking spaces in the same building, adverse health effects for the occupants of the smoking room cannot be controlled by ventilation. No other engineering approaches, including current and advanced dilution ventilation or air-cleaning technologies, have been demonstrated or should be relied on to control health risks from ETS exposure in spaces where smoking occurs. Some engineering measures may reduce that exposure and the corresponding risk to some degree while also addressing to some extent the comfort issues of odor and some forms of irritation. An increasing number of local and national governments, as well as

many private building owners, are implementing bans on indoor smoking. Because of ASHRAE's mission to act for the benefit of the public, it encourages elimination of smoking in the indoor environment as the optimal way to minimize ETS exposure.

How much ventilation or air cleaning would it require to create an acceptable health risk for workers in an establishment under typical conditions of smoking? For a typical bar in the state of Delaware, with a smoking prevalence of 23 percent (or an average of 2.7 cigarettes being smoked constantly per 100 cubic meters of volume), I calculated that the amount to achieve the same effect as a smoking ban, the ventilation rate would have to be increased 22,500-fold, amounting to 121,500 air changes per hour, which would require an indoor tornado (Repace, 2005).

Indoor versus Outdoor Air Pollution

The assertion that secondhand smoke poses less exposure to air pollution than automobile traffic is unjustified. First, most vehicles have long been subject to strict emission controls in the United States, with harmful substances, such as lead, banned from gasoline, and catalytic converters used to reduce carbon monoxide and hydrocarbon emissions. Second, cigarettes are exempt from emission controls. Third, tobacco smoke makes far worse respirable particulate (RSP) pollution than traffic (Repace, 2004; Repace and Lowrey, 1980)—this was true in the days before catalytic converters and is even truer today. After Delaware enacted a statewide smoke-free workplace law, the measured concentration of toxic and carcinogenic air pollutants in a casino, six bars, and a pool hall decreased by 85–95 percent (Repace, 2004). Prior to the smoking ban, all venues were heavily polluted, with indoor respirable particle (RSP) levels averaging 20 times outdoor background. For workers, these levels violated the National Ambient Air Quality Standard for fine particulate matter by a factor of nearly five. Delaware hospitality workers were exposed to RSP levels far higher than on city streets heavily polluted by truck and bus traffic. Before the ban, indoor carcinogens in Delaware averaged five times higher than outdoor background levels, tripling workers' daily exposure and exceeding the highest levels of carcinogens measured at an interstate tollbooth at the traffic-choked Baltimore Harbor Tunnel.

Secondhand smoke kills. There is no justification for exposing workers or the public to this toxic agent. It cannot be controlled by ventilation or air cleaning, and arguments of economic losses to business are not supported by data and unfairly exclude the economic and health losses to workers from this toxic exposure. Businesses must honor their obligation to provide a safe and healthy workplace for their workers and their customers and not be held hostage to unsubstantiated fears of economic decline. Arguments to maintain smoking in hospitality venues are really arguments in favor of preserving smoking for a new generation of nicotine addicts.

REFERENCES

Biener, L., and Fitzgerald, G. 1999. Smoky bars and restaurants: who avoids them and why? *Journal of Public Health Management and Practice* 5:74–78.

California Department of Health Services, Tobacco Control Section. 2001. *Eliminating Smoking in Bars, Taverns, and Gaming Clubs: The California Smoke-Free Workplace Act.* Sacramento: California Department of Health Services.

California Department of Health Services, Tobacco Control Section. 2004. California Tobacco Control Update, 2004. Sacramento: California Department of Health Services.

Mandel, L. L., Alamar, B. C., and Glantz, S. A. 2005. Delaware smoke-free law did not affect revenue from gaming. *Tobacco Control Online* 14:10–12. http://tc.bmj.com/cgi/content/full/14/1/10.

New York City Department of Finance, New York City Department of Health and Mental Hygiene, New York City Department of Small Business Services, New York City Economic Development Corporation. 2004. *The State of Smoke-Free New York City: A One-Year Review.* New York: New York City Department of Health and Mental Hygiene.

Novick, L. F. 1999. From the editor. *Journal of Public Health Management and Practice* 5:v.

Repace, J. L. 2004. Respirable particles and carcinogens in the air of Delaware hospitality venues before and after a smoking ban. *Journal of Occupational and Environmental Medicine* 46:887–905.

Repace, J. L. 2005. Controlling tobacco smoke pollution: technical feature. *ASHRAE IAQ Applications* 6 (3):11–15.

Repace, J. L., Jinot, J., Bayard, S., Emmons, K., and Hammond, S. K. 1998. Air nicotine and saliva cotinine as indicators of passive smoking exposure and risk. *Risk Analysis* 18:71–83.

Repace, J. L., and Lowrey, A. H. 1980. Indoor air pollution, tobacco smoke, and public health. *Science* 208 (4443):464–72.

U.S. Environmental Protection Agency. 1997. *The Benefits and Costs of the Clean Air Act, 1970–1990.* 410-R-97–002. Washington, D.C.: U.S. Environmental Protection Agency.

25

The Role of the Food and Drug Administration in Accelerating the Development and Release of New Medications for the Addictions

CURTIS WRIGHT, M.D., M.P.H.

The cost of developing new drugs has risen to approximately $400–800 million per drug approved (DiMasi et al., 2003). To make development of a new product feasible, a firm must anticipate a profit on sales exceeding this figure. To make such an investment, drug development companies must find a situation in which either their new medication will provide a return far greater than the average (i.e., a "blockbuster" drug) or the costs of development will be far less than average.

It is not known whether the high cost of drug development is due to the difficulty and expense of needed research or the expense of complying with ever-increasing international and domestic regulations, guidances, and rules governing the development, testing, manufacture, reimbursement, and sale of pharmaceuticals (Office of Technology Assessment, 1993). Driven by ever-improving systems for collecting data on adverse events associated with pharmacotherapy, a low societal tolerance of adverse events, and concerns about prescription drug safety, the U.S. Food and Drug Administration (FDA) strives to ensure that medications are as safe as possible and effective in use. The agency's focus on safety at all costs may be a significant contributor to the continuing upward spiral of development costs (U.S. Department of Health and Human Services, 2005).

Regulatory Obstacles to the Development of New Pharmaceuticals

During the late twentieth century, "generic" drug regulations were established with the intent of correcting the tendency of the costs of the development and approval process to create barriers to developing new products (U.S. Congress, Office of Technology Assessment, 1993). This allowed generic firms to make and sell a copy of a new drug without incurring the development costs faced by the innovator drug, thus providing new drugs at a cheaper price to the patient but markedly reducing the financial return to the innovator.

The result was predictable. Pharmaceutical firms must direct scarce development dollars either to products that have a large potential population of patients or to products for serious diseases for which high prices will willingly be paid (or both). Treatments for conditions not meeting these criteria are unattractive investments, and certain disorders (where revenues were low because the at-risk population was small) were effectively "orphaned." Regulations governing "orphan" drugs were put in place to provide additional incentives for rare disorders (U.S. Department of Health and Human Services, 1992), but no provisions were made within the FDA to promote development of drugs for conditions that are not rare but are common among patients who rely on publicly funded health care rather than private health insurance. This has significant implications for substance abuse treatment because there are few incentives for pharmaceutical development of drugs where the predicted profit from an eventually marketed product would be less than the costs of development.

Most substance abuse treatment programs are publicly funded. Because treatment funding is under continuous cost containment pressure, it has not (yet) offered the prospect of sufficient financial return to make investment in this area attractive to the pharmaceutical industry (Institute of Medicine [IOM], 1995). Some efforts were made by government to address this problem. Medications development groups were established within several National Institutes of Health (Public Law 100–690, 1988)—the National Institute on Drug Abuse (NIDA), National Institute on Alcohol Abuse and Alcoholism (NIAAA), and National Institute of Mental Health (NIMH)—but these efforts were in large part frustrated by the basic economics of the problem. A review of the situation by the IOM in 1995 led it to conclude that coordinated efforts at the federal level were needed if any new medications for the addictive diseases were to be developed (IOM, 1995).

The dilemma was simple: either there had to be a provision for increasing the revenue potential for these products, or the costs of developing them had to be reduced, or both. One such strategy was developed in pediatrics. Many of the medications used in pediatrics were never studied for safety or effectiveness in pediatric populations. To address this problem, the FDA established a program that mandated the study of new drugs in pediatric populations. To help offset industry's costs of carrying out the required studies, the agency allowed for near-term patent extension of existing drugs (thus improving financial return) if study of such drugs was needed in children (U.S. Department of Health and Human Services, 2000).

Although this program was successful in promoting testing of successful adult drugs in pediatric populations, it did little to prompt the development of new drugs specific to children's needs (U.S. Department of Health and Human Services, 2002). Hence the Best Pharmaceuticals for Children Act, which is intended to encourage broader assessment of drugs used in pediatric populations, was signed into law January 4, 2002 (Public Law 107–109, 2002).

Another program established in the 1990s sought to reduce development costs by making it easier for medications development groups within the NIH to bring new drugs to the review divisions at the FDA (U.S. Department of Health and Human Services, 1989; U.S. General Accounting Office, 1994). This program was initially quite successful in stimulating research through cooperative agreements between the medications development groups and the pharmaceutical industry, but as we enter the twenty-first century it is not clear that it is continuing to achieve its intended purpose. Whether that is due to organizational changes within the FDA or to other factors is not clear.

At present, policies are not working to stimulate the development of new treatments for the addictions, but the blame does not necessarily lie completely (if at all) with the government. The empowering legislation for the FDA had its roots in the sanitary reform movements of the early 1900s, a time when the task of government was to prevent and correct corrupt business practices that endangered the public. With rare exceptions, such as for life-threatening diseases, the machinery of pharmaceutical regulation is aimed at restraining, not encouraging, industry, and few regulations actually aim at facilitating the development of new medications (U.S. Department of Health and Human Services, 1992, 2000). This is due, in part, to the potential conflict of interest inherent in having the individuals who assess the risk of a treatment working as advocates for the development of that treatment (U.S. Department of Health and Human Services, 2005).

Sociological Obstacles to New Treatments for Substance Abuse

Perhaps a more important factor in the failure to develop new medications for substance abuse than these regulatory obstacles is the fact that our culture does not take substance abuse disorders seriously, despite a lethality and societal cost that makes them the leading cause of death, disability, and loss of productive years of life in the United States. Disorders involving tobacco, alcohol, and narcotics (both illicit drugs and diverted prescription medications) are associated with astronomical morbidity and mortality rates (IOM, 1995). Perhaps as much as 10 percent of children who experiment with drugs and alcohol have an established addictive disorder by high school, and many people have developed multiple concurrent substance abuse problems by the third decade of life (Substance Abuse and Mental Health Services Administration [SAMHSA], 2004). It is unfortunate that the natural social forces of control in the adolescent and young adult years depend on stigmatization to control abuse of these agents. Stigmatizing abuse to reduce the risk of first use results in a tendency either to resist the concept of treatment, to stigmatize those in treatment, or, paradoxically, to stimulate abuse among some adolescents. In some social sectors and settings there is a reluctance to recognize, fund, accept, or permit intervention and treatment.

Although society at large may consider injury from addiction to be the "just desserts" of drug abuse, this perspective is not shared by those responsible for the public health. From the public health perspective, the path forward is to recognize and accept that these disorders are a major public health problem, that they cluster together as a diagnosis and cannot be treated in isolation from each other, and that they afflict a large percentage of the population, including adolescents. Change is possible, however, and the FDA can help accomplish this while remaining within its mandate.

A great deal of addiction treatment is provided outside of conventional office-based medical practice. Much of the treatment for alcohol or tobacco use is provided in self-care models, such as Alcoholics Anonymous or over-the-counter nicotine-replacement products. Methadone clinics, which provide one form of substitution treatment, the most effective therapy for opioid dependence, are among the most highly regulated outpatient practices in medicine. Substitution treatment with buprenorphine is less tightly regulated, but, whereas physicians are now allowed to prescribe buprenorphine for addiction in office practice, relatively few (as a percentage) have been certified to do so (SAMHSA Buprenorphine Physician Locator).

For whatever reason, there are few physicians or medical institutions to speak to the need for addiction treatment. Many of the clinical experts and clinical researchers in this area were trained almost 40 years ago, and relatively few physicians are currently entering the field. The lack of strong physician advocates has been one of the factors leading to why the FDA treats these disorders as lower priority illnesses than many other diseases. Thus, for example, the FDA has applied fast-track approval strategies to cancer and HIV treatment but not to treatments for the cigarette smoking and intravenous drug abuse that often lead to those diseases. Most of the oversight of research, development, review, and approval of addiction treatment medicines has been assigned to divisions within the agency whose major and priority task is the review of commercial neuropharmacologic agents, analgesics, or anesthetics and that have relatively little expertise in addiction medicine. As a consequence, experts in the field rarely oversee the primary reviews of drugs for the treatment of these disorders. It is extremely difficult for the FDA to recruit, train, and retain review staff in general and harder still to recruit and retain those with actual treatment experience or expertise in either addiction medicine or in pharmaceutical development. This has been exacerbated in recent years by excessive turnover in review staff and legislative and budgetary restrictions that have led to the disbanding of the FDA Drug Abuse Advisory Committee, a group of external experts called on to advise the agency in this area (U.S. Department of Health and Human Services, 2001). The overall situation, then, is that current FDA structure does not facilitate the development of drugs for the treatment of addictions in any substantive fashion, and the political sensitivity of these products and disorders act to make these products controversial, further restricting development in this area.

There Is a Path Forward

The first helpful action to enable FDA to better facilitate bringing addiction treatments to market would be to convene a Public Health Service (PHS) Task Force charged to produce a comprehensive White Paper or Surgeon General's Report on addiction. Such a document would address the epidemiology of these disorders (tobacco, alcohol, and drugs), the initiation in the school years, clustering of diagnoses, and the burden of morbidity and mortality both among young adults and later in life. It would thus bring public attention to the burdens that these disorders as a group impose on our educational, criminal justice, health care, and public health systems, as well as employment.

In addition, the surgeon general or other appropriate PHS official should make a determination that the addictive disorders are serious and life-threatening illnesses for which current therapy is unsatisfactory. This would allow priority review at the FDA, which in turn should establish a division of addiction research and addiction drug products whose clinical staff must all have credible clinical experience treating substance abuse and dependence to review research activities involving drugs of abuse and regulation of products for the addictions to tobacco, alcohol, and other drugs.

In its 1992 report, the IOM criticized the FDA advisory committee structure, which is still in place, noting that agency control over the number, composition, membership, and agenda of its advisory committees rendered them ineffective as a source of medical and scientific peer review on which to base agency actions (Rettig et al., 1992). The PHS should address the major gap in FDA's current structure by establishing an advisory committee in keeping with the IOM's recommendations, that is, a committee that includes representation from the NIH institutes most involved with the addictions (NIDA, NIAAA, NIMH, the National Cancer Institute, and the National Heart, Lung, and Blood Institute) and the Centers for Disease Control and Prevention, in addition to physicians in the field. If the FDA division managing addiction drug products had to openly discuss its actions (or inaction) on pending applications with those tasked with developing new science and managing these disorders, the result would be a more fruit-ful process.

If this is to happen, the PHS must help develop the next generation of experts in addiction medicine. It must promote one or more pro-grams specifically to attract, train, and develop clinicians with expert-ise in treating addictions within the PHS and government service in general and to make those physicians accessible to the FDA. In light of the high cost of medical education, student loan reimbursement pro-grams coupled with extramural training (highly effective in the past) could be reinstated. It is a simple fact, known to the FDA, that effec-tive review staff in all scientific disciplines (medicine, pharmacology, chemistry, pharmacokinetics, and statistics) must not only be expert in their discipline but must also have hands-on clinical expertise.

These recommendations outline a strategy for reducing the costs of developing new treatments for the addictions by improving the regu-latory process. They will not be effective unless bold measures are also taken to address the problem of marginal revenues for these products.

As stated above, the overarching problem is that drug discovery can-didates are not being brought into development because the net pres-ent value (the worth of future revenues in today's dollars minus costs of development) is too low for developers to make a profit. This is the one area where the FDA can take unilateral action with relative ease, adapting the treatment investigational new drug (IND) process as it did previously to make methadone available for treatment (U.S. De-partment of Health, Education and Welfare, 1970).

There is a provision in the FDA regulations (21 CFR 312.7) that allows a commercial sponsor to charge for an investigational drug either directly or under a treatment IND, provided such charges do not exceed the properly accounted costs of research, development, manu-facture, and handling of the investigational drug. Using this provision would enable a firm to generate a cash flow that would improve the net present value and profitability of the project. Most firms do not use this provision, because it requires that they demonstrate to the FDA that the price charged for the investigational drug does not exceed their costs. Most firms' accounting systems are not organized to support the required project-by-project audit, and the anxiety attendant on such an event acts as a powerful disincentive.

It would take little for the FDA to decide that there are certain indi-cations, conditions, and therapeutic areas, such as drug abuse or addiction, for which such requests for reimbursement would be accepted or encouraged. With a little facilitation by the relevant NIH Institutes and the IOM, this might allow more products to jump the development gap into clinical use and put more compounds into the development pipelines.

Increasing the net present value of products in development will be in the interests of public health only if it can be shown that this is an area in which the potential profits to companies have been inadequate to support new drug development. Those familiar with the process are all too aware that this is the case. To date, no new medications for the treatment of alcoholism or illicit drug addiction have proved to be commercially successful.

REFERENCES

DiMasi, J.A., Hansen, R.W., and Grabowski, H.G. 2003. The price of innovation: new estimates of drug development costs. *Journal of Health Economics* 22:151–85.

Institute of Medicine. 1995. *The Development of Medications for the Treatment of Opiate and Cocaine Addictions: Issues for the Government and Private Sector.* Washington D.C.: National Academy Press.

Public Law 100–690. 1988. The Drug-Free Workplace Act. http://uscode .house.gov/download/pls/41C10.txt.

Public Law 107–109. 2002. The Best Pharmaceuticals for Children Act. www.fda.gov/cder/pediatric/PL107–109.pdf.

Rettig, R. A., Earley, L. E., and Merrill, R. A., eds. 1992. *Food and Drug Administration Advisory Committees, Committee to Study the Use of Advisory Committees by the Food and Drug Administration, Institute of Medicine.* Washington, D.C.: National Academy Press.

Substance Abuse and Mental Health Services Administration Data. 2000. Buprenorphine Physician Locator. SAMHSA, U.S. Department of Health and Human Services. www.buprenorphine.samhsa.gov.

Substance Abuse and Mental Health Services Administration, Office of Applied Studies. 2004. *Results from the 2003 National Household Survey on Drug Abuse: National Findings.* Office of Applied Studies, NSDUH Series H-25, DHHS Publication No. (SMA) 04–3964. Rockville, Md.: U.S. Department of Health and Human Services.

U.S. Congress, Office of Technology Assessment. 1993. *Pharmaceutical R&D: Costs, Risks, and Rewards.* OTA-H-522. Washington, D.C.: Government Printing Office, pp. 136–38. www.wws.princeton.edu/~ota/ ns20/alpha f.html.

U.S. Department of Health and Human Services. 1992. 21 CFR Part 316; Orphan Drug Act. Revised April 2004. www.fda.gov/orphan/oda.htm.

U.S. Department of Health and Human Services. 2005. Draft guidance for industry on the Food and Drug Administration's "Drug Watch" for emerging drug safety information. Docket no. 2005D-0062, *Federal Register* 70, no 89 (May 10): 24606–607.

U.S. Department of Health, Education, and Welfare, Food and Drug Administration. 1970. 21 CFR Part 130, Conditions for investigational use of methadone for maintenance programs for addicts. *Federal Register* 35, 110.113, June 11, 1970, pp. 9014–16.

U.S. Department of Health and Human Services, Food and Drug Administration. 1989. Pilot Drug Review Division. www.fda.gov/bbs/topics/ANSWERS/ANS00169.html.

U.S. Department of Health and Human Services, Food and Drug Administration. 1992. Orphan Drug Act. www.fda.gov/orphan/oda.htm: 21 CFR Part 316. Docket 85N-AB55.

U.S. Department of Health and Human Services, Food and Drug Administration. 2002. Obtaining timely pediatric studies of and adequate pediatric labeling for human drugs and biologies. Docket 02N-0152. www.fda.gov/cber/rules/pedlabel.htm.

U.S. Department of Health and Human Services, Food and Drug Administration. 2005. Draft Guidance for Industry on the Food and Drug Administration's "Drug Watch" for Emerging Drug Safety Information; Availability. Docket 2005D-0062, *Federal Register* 70 (89): 24606–607.

U.S. Department of Health and Human Services, Food and Drug Administration, Center for Drug Evaluation and Research, Center for Biologics Evaluation and Research. 2000. Guidance for Industry. Recommendations for Complying with the Pediatric Rule (21 CFR 314.55[a] and 601.27[a]). www.fda.gov/cber/gdlns/pedrule.pdf.

U.S. Department of Health and Human Services, Food and Drug Administration, Center for Drug Evaluation and Research, Center for Biologics Evaluation and Research. 2001. Woodcock, J., Drug Abuse Advisory Committee. Letter, April 6. www.fda.gov/cder/audiences/acspage/daac-letter.htm.

U.S. General Accounting Office. 1994. FDA User fees. Current measures not sufficient for evaluating effect. http://archive.qao.gov/d14t3/152382.pdf.

26

Smoking Status as the New Vital Sign
Progress and Challenges

Michael C. Fiore, M.D., M.P.H.

At the beginning of the twentieth century, the model of "vital signs," now a well-known clinical assessment tool, was introduced to confront infectious disease, the leading cause of death at that time. Vital signs included temperature, pulse, respiratory rate, and, later, blood pressure. Today vital signs are essential to how clinicians evaluate, diagnose, and treat patients. Now virtually every patient who presents to a health care setting in the United States has his or her vital signs checked, usually before the clinician examines the patient.

At the beginning of the twenty-first century, tobacco use is the leading cause of preventable death in the United States (Minino et al., 2002). Perhaps the most promising (and realistic) first step to reduce tobacco use in our time would be to add smoking status to the catalogue of vital signs (Figure 26.1).

The singularly devastating health impact of cigarette smoking is all the warrant needed to make this fundamental change in the way health care is delivered. Since it was proposed as a vital sign in 1991 (Fiore, 1991), determining the patient's smoking status has become the standard of care in many clinics across the United States, but it is not yet a universal practice. Yet as with the other vital signs, the data suggest that the simple institutional change of eliciting information relating to tobacco use leads clinicians to change their clinical practice: when smoking status is added to the vital signs, clinicians are

VITAL SIGNS

Blood Pressure:_____

Pulse:_____ **Weight:**_____

Temperature:_____

Respiratory Rate:_____

Tobacco Use: Current   Former   Never (circle one)

Figure 26.1. Tobacco status added to vital signs assessment

more likely to advise smokers to quit and encourage former smokers to stay quit (Fiore, 1991; Fiore et al., 1995).

Like checking blood pressure or temperature, assessing smoking status opens the door to enlisting patients in a major disease prevention effort. Patients rarely object to having their blood pressure monitored at clinic visits, and there are no data to suggest that they would object to regular assessment of smoking status. In fact, recent research suggests the opposite—that patients have come to expect clinicians to pay some attention to their smoking status (Gallup Organization, 1999; Cluss and Moss, 2002; Solberg et al., 2001). Acting on such data, physicians and other clinicians can treat patients who smoke, offer support to patients who have quit, and help patients deal with episodes of relapse, a common feature of this addictive, chronic disease.

A Simple Strategy That Works

More than 70 percent of smokers see a physician each year, but fewer than two-thirds of these patients recall being asked about their smoking status (Cokkinides et al., 2005). Including smoking status as a vital sign is a simple yet fundamental change in clinical practice, but one that has enormous potential for public health. An early, prospective study of the effect of expanding the vital signs to include smoking showed a dramatic rise in the number of patients (from 58 percent to

81 percent) who recalled being asked about their smoking (Fiore et al., 1995).

Once smoking status is documented, clinicians have a prime opportunity to assist patients in a behavior change that will improve their health and quality of life and can add as many as 14 years of potential life. Approximately 70 percent of all smokers acknowledge that they want to quit, and physician advice to do so is an important motivator in getting patients started. Evidence shows that even two to three minutes of physician counseling can substantially increase the likelihood that a smoker will successfully quit (U.S. Preventive Services Task Force, 2003).

Assuring that clinicians document smoking status as a vital sign is relatively easy and costfree. Vital signs are almost ubiquitously recorded and can be documented by clinic or hospital support personnel. When patient smoking status is identified this way, clinicians are free to focus on an appropriate means of intervention for each smoker.

Why is so simple a change taking so long to implement? It has taken the better part of 15 years to whittle away at the myths about smoking and about patient attitudes that keep many clinicians from adopting the smoking status vital sign:

Myth: Patients will object to being counseled about quitting.

Fact: Research indicates the opposite. Patients believe it is within the physician's purview to address their smoking and often expect it (Gallup Organization, 1999; Cluss and Moss, 2002; Solberg et al., 2001).

Myth: Clinicians are not prepared to counsel patients about quitting and to follow through with the necessary actions—planning a quit date, offering evidence-based pharmacotherapies and motivational counseling, arranging follow-up to forestall or prevent relapse.

Fact: Guidance or instruction in smoking cessation counseling is now widely available in many forms, including Web-based, and can be quickly learned and applied (Carpenter et al., 2003).

Myth: Because of the significant relapse rate, assisting patients in quitting smoking seems a fruitless endeavor.

Fact: A patient who attempts to quit "cold turkey" with no assistance at all is the one not likely to succeed, and "cold turkey" is the method currently employed by approximately 80 percent of the 20 million smokers who try to quit each year (Gallup Organization, 1999). Evidence shows that medication, counseling, and follow-up support provided by a clinician can minimize relapse episodes and greatly increase successful abstinence (Fiore et al., 1995; U.S. Preventive Services Task Force, 2003).

How Do We Get There from Here?

If current trends regarding tobacco use continue, we will not be able to achieve the Healthy People 2010 goal of reducing smoking prevalence in the United States to 12 percent. Implementing smoking status as a universal vital sign for all patients is a crucial first step in our effort, but it is not sufficient in itself. If we are to increase significantly the rates at which physicians intervene in their patients' smoking, we must remind physicians of the immense power they have to influence the health behavior of Americans. Physicians in this country still have the logistical and moral force to confront the epidemic of tobacco addiction, illness, and death.

Decades from now, treatment for tobacco dependence will benefit from emerging research on new pharmacotherapies, relapse interventions, and insights into the addictive process. Integrating documentation of smoking status into the regular delivery of health care as a "systems change" has the potential to reach the more than 30 million smokers who visit primary care physicians each year. Decades from now, when tobacco use is a truly uncommon behavior, institutional changes such as expanding the vital signs to include smoking status will be recognized as one of the key approaches that contributed to this public health success.

REFERENCES

Carpenter, K.M., Watson, J.M., and Raffety, B. 2003. Teaching brief interventions for smoking cessation via an interactive computer-based tutorial. *Journal of Health Psychology* 8:149–60.

Cluss, P.A., and Moss, D. 2002. Parent attitudes about pediatricians addressing parental smoking. *Ambulatory Pediatrics* 2:485–88.

Cokkinides, V.E., Ward, E., Jemal, A., and Thun, M.J. 2005. Under-use of smoking-cessation treatments: results from the National Health Interview Survey, 2000. *American Journal of Preventive Medicine* 28:119–22.

Fiore, M.C. 1991. The new vital sign: assessing and documenting smoking status. *JAMA* 266:3183–85.

Fiore, M.C., Jorenby, D.E., Schensky, A.E., Smith, S.S., Bauer, R.R., and Baker, T.B. 1995. Smoking status as the new vital sign: effect on assessment and intervention in patients who smoke. *Mayo Clinic Proceedings* 70:209–13.

Gallup Organization: 1999. *Attitudes and Behaviors Related to Smoking Cessation.* New York: Gallup Organization.

Minino, A.M., Arias, E., Kochanek, K.D., Murphy, S.L., and Smith, B.L. 2002. Deaths: final data for 2000. *National Vital Statistics Report* 50:1–119.

Solberg, L.I., Boyle, R.G., Davidson, G., Magnan, S.J., and Carlson, C.L. 2001. Patient satisfaction and discussion of smoking cessation during clinical visits. *Mayo Clinic Proceedings* 76:138–43.

U.S. Preventive Services Task Force. 2003. *Counseling to Prevent Tobacco Use and Tobacco-Caused Disease: Recommendation Statement.* Rockville, Md.: Agency for Healthcare Research and Quality.

Epilogue

JACK E. HENNINGFIELD, PH.D.,
PATRICIA B. SANTORA, PH.D., AND
WARREN K. BICKEL, PH.D.

As the foregoing chapters reveal, the state of addiction treatment in the United States has much in common with the lives of many addicted individuals. Like the lives of persons with addictions, addiction treatment is in disarray; it does not have a clear path and offers alternative courses that are daunting in their complexity. There is little apparent consensus among the experts. The issues span nomenclature, theoretical perspective, diagnostic concerns and determining appropriate treatment interventions.

Additional complications are raised by the diversity of problems posed by the range of drugs of abuse, which differ radically in effect and pattern of use, as well as by the diversity of substance abusers. Can significant commonalities be found in the needs and appropriate interventions for diverse subpopulations of "substance abusers" that include pregnant women who use intravenous drugs, young men who abuse methamphetamine, youth who smoke cigarettes, adults who abuse alcohol, people of all ages who smoke marijuana, and those who abuse prescription drugs? Never has H. L. Mencken's comment been so apropos, "For every complex problem there is a solution that is simple, neat, and wrong."

The chapters in this volume show clearly that there are no simple, neat, or easy solutions to the problem of substance abuse and addiction. They reinforce the conclusion of addiction science pioneer Avram Goldstein, who argued, "Like all public-health problems, addiction is a complex one, with multiple causes, multiple prevention strategies, and multiple cures" (2001, p. 3). To address addiction as a public health problem, he proposed "drug-by-drug policies." The present contributors take a step further and argue for a portfolio approach to drug treatment in which drug-by-drug, population-by-population policies provide a means to address the enormous public health challenge of substance abuse and addiction.

The challenge is formidable. Substance abuse and addiction have reached epidemic levels. They are among the most prevalent, deadly, and costly health problems in the United States today, appear prominently among the leading causes of death, and are major contributors to heart disease, cancer, and stroke. Each year, patients whose presenting illnesses are severely complicated by substance abuse and addiction fill U.S. hospitals. Patients with co-occurring substance abuse and addiction do not adhere adequately to prescribed medical care and have poor treatment outcomes, increased hospitalizations, and increased costs. As we noted in our preface to this volume, the economic effects of substance abuse and addiction are enormous, with the combined costs of health care, lost productivity, and crime estimated at well over one-half trillion U.S. dollars. Appropriate interventions are urgently needed to improve the quality of care, control substance abuse and addiction, and reduce health care costs.

Leading addiction scientists have reached an "unsettling consensus" that our society has no organized system of care to meet the treatment needs of those with substance abuse and addiction problems. In fact, as Alan Leshner notes in chapter 17, major gaps persist between what research has shown to be effective and what is actually practiced in clinical settings. Those gaps are beginning to be addressed. For example, the Institute of Medicine's newly released report, *Improving the Quality of Health Care for Mental and Substance-Use Conditions* (2006), offers recommendations for addressing the unmet health care needs of those with substance abuse and addiction and its co-occurrence with other medical and psychiatric disorders. Similarly, the provocative and timely book, *Rethinking Substance Abuse: What the Science Shows, and What We Should Do about It* (2006), edited by addiction treatment scientists William R. Miller and Kathleen M. Carroll, provides a coherent set of much-needed guidelines for building better systems of care. By acknowledging the need for an organized system of care to address substance abuse and addiction problems and arguing for interventions based on scientific knowledge rather than opinion or ideology, these volumes lay a solid foundation for addressing the complex needs of individuals with substance abuse and addiction problems.

Acknowledging substance abuse and addiction as public health problems argues for improving our ability to monitor rapidly the course, nature, and prevalence of abuse and addiction. Compare our ability to track annual influenza cycles, HIV/AIDS transmission, and outbreaks of bacterial disease to our slow-to-respond national surveillance systems on substance abuse and addiction, which often lag several years behind in documenting trends. Likewise, acknowledging substance abuse and addiction as public health problems opens the door to using a diversity of approaches to meet the many distinct needs posed by different populations and the numerous ways disease is expressed. Conceiving substance abuse and addiction as public health problems also brings with it the recognition that all are best served when prevention efforts work hand in hand with treatment efforts, each mutually supportive, each contributing to overall reduction in prevalence of disease and reduction in adverse consequences when disease does occur. Finally, understanding substance abuse and addiction as public health problems can help us put into play broad education and communications programs for laypersons, health care professionals, and policymakers. To reach our diverse society, communications efforts must range from scientific publications, to newspaper articles, to Internet sites, to art.

The chapters in this volume offer insight, guidance, and hope born of some rather surprising points of consensus. Three key consensus points emerge from these chapters: however we view it, substance abuse and addiction require treatment; stigma is a potent force; and substance abuse and addiction are pervasive in society.

First, treatment is essential. Whether substance abuse and addiction are best viewed as "disease," "disorder," "voluntary behavior," or "psychosocial display," there are individuals whose drug use is not within their control and who need and can benefit from some sort of intervention, which we prefer to call "treatment." This is obvious to professionals working in the addictions field, but the prevailing view among individuals suffering with addictions, and among lay persons as well, is that controlling addiction is simply a matter of "determination," "willpower," "prayer," or "motivation." Without denying that each of these holds promise, at least for some, we are more convinced than ever that providing treatment for persons with substance abuse disorders is legitimate and vital.

Second, stigma is powerful. At first glance, it might seem that irreconcilable perspectives have emerged about stigma and drug abuse. Some chapters argued strongly that stigmatization is destructive and inhibits individuals from acknowledging problematic substance use and seeking treatment. Others argued just as compellingly that stigmatization provides an environmental pressure to stop drug abuse, seek treatment, and remain abstinent; however, we see common ground here. In our view, neither "side" was arguing that substance abusers should not have to take responsibility for or admit the harmfulness of their behavior, nor was either side arguing against the view that substance abuse is undesirable and harmful to the individual abuser and others. As we see it, both perspectives can converge in the view that we should treat substance abusers with respect and dignity by offering them treatment and by making every effort to reinforce the view that substance abuse and addiction harm everyone. This is consistent with Dr. Koop's recommendation that we "fight the disease of addiction and the purveyors of disease, not those afflicted."

Finally, substance abuse and addiction permeate the entire fabric of our society. No population is immune. Anyone can be adversely affected by the addiction of friends and loved ones, as well as unknown persons. If we accept and support this view, we should be more willing as individuals and as a nation to vigorously tackle this public health challenge.

Substance abuse and addiction have reached epidemic proportions and demand vigorous action as urgent public health problems. By starting from a scientific knowledge base on the problematic use of tobacco, alcohol, and other drugs and exploring the clinical implications for treatment and prevention, our nation can develop strategies that will reduce and control addiction, just as it did for other seemingly intractable public health challenges, such as polio, smallpox, and HIV/AIDS. The chapters in this book provide grist for vigorous debate, and we hope they will stimulate renewed commitment that will revolutionize the state of drug addiction treatment in the twenty-first century.

REFERENCES

Goldstein A. 2001. *Addiction: From Biology to Drug Policy.* New York: Oxford University Press.

Institute of Medicine of the National Academies. 2006. *Improving the Quality of Health Care for Mental and Substance-Use Conditions.* Washington, D.C.: National Academies Press.

Miller, W.R., and Carroll, K.M., eds. 2006. *Rethinking Substance Abuse: What the Science Shows, and What We Should Do about It.* New York: Guilford Press.

Index